Connect the Docs
Put Digital Health into Practice

A Handbook for Clinicians

Edited by Jared Johnson

First edition, November 2016.

Copyright © 2016 Ultera Digital LLC.
www.ulteradigital.com

All rights reserved.
Except as permitted under U.S. Copyright Act of 1976,
no part of this publication may be reproduced, distributed,
transmitted in any form or by any means, or stored in a
database or retrieval system, without prior written permission.

ISBN-10: 1539358933
ISBN-13: 978-1539358930

*For the health IT community and clinicians everywhere
who are using digital health to revolutionize patient care.*

*For Stephanie, Dallin, Alexa, Lance and Kiera,
who support me every time I say, "I've got a big idea."*

*In memory of Lenard, whose life was spent in service,
and whose early death inspires me to make health care better.*

Ad astra per aspera.

CONTENTS

	Acknowledgments	9
	Introduction	10

SECTION I: PARTNERING WITH PATIENTS

1	**It Doesn't Take More Time** Danny Sands, MD	15
2	**Silence Can Be Catastrophic** Farris Timimi, MD	25
3	**We Can't Know All the Answers** Wendy Sue Swanson, MD	35
4	**Partner With Patients** "e-Patient Dave" deBronkart	45
5	**You Can't Complain About Bad Content If You Aren't Creating Good Content** Justin Smith, MD	53
6	**Patient Satisfaction Scores Affect Reimbursement Rates** Mandi Bishop	63
7	**Create Highly Engaged Patients and Families** Tanya Altmann, MD	69

8	**Position Digital Marketing Experts to Lead** Aaron Watkins	79
9	**Build an Online Community** John Lynn	85
10	**Health Care is Always Personal** Linda Stotsky	93

SECTION II: USING DIGITAL HEALTH TOOLS

11	**The Early Adopter Advantage** Wen Dombrowki, MD and Fard Johnmar	101
12	**Reduce the Barriers to Entry** Richard Milani, MD	109
13	**Tame the Data Beast** Rasu Shrestha, MD	115
14	**Create Behavioral Change** Matt Patterson, MD	125
15	**Patient Engagement Changes the Game** Sterling Lanier	131
16	**Focus on Current Patients, Not Just New Ones** Shawn Gross	139
17	**Play Nice With the CIO** David Chou	147

18	**Own Your Career** Sue Schade	153
19	**Collaboration is the New Success** Nick Adkins	159
	About the Author	163

ACKNOWLEDGMENTS

I recently heard Dr. Roni Zeiger, the former chief health strategist at Google, give a keynote where he described the end of the era where one person comes up with the perfect idea. The new economy of ideas is highly collaborative, he explained, in a way that can be more powerful than anything previously designed in isolation.

To that end, this book shows off the willingness of the health care community to join forces for the sake of better ideas. It is the collaborative wisdom of dozens of podcast guests and thought leaders, many of whose words cannot be included simply due to space but who have happily contributed ideas and experiences along the way. This is a result of the collective consciousness of an industry that is poised for revolution. As Dr. Zeiger put it, one person may know more than any of us, but surely they can't know more than *all* of us.

INTRODUCTION

A year ago I set out to answer the question, "How can clinicians put digital health into practice?"

At the time I had my own digital marketing consulting agency with clients in the provider, health IT and technology spaces. I was observing the innovation going on in health IT. The *democratization of medicine*, as Dr. Eric Topol put it. Remote monitoring apps syncing with smartphones via Bluetooth. Patient-generated health data transmitted from Apple Watches. Live video streaming of surgeries on Periscope. Genomic and proteomic research fueling personalized chemotherapy cocktails in real time.

This is light years beyond yesterday's medicine. And a critical mass of today's clinicians—including many of you reading this book—now have overcome any initial resistance. You know tomorrow's health care is only scratching the surface. So now what?

By mid-2015 I heard a lot of voices demanding that physicians adopt digital health tools, but few, if any, of those voices explained what to do and how to do it, in ways that physicians relate to. What did I do about it? As a digital engagement evangelist, I turned to content marketing. I launched a weekly podcast called Health IT Marketer and started interviewing those who had discovered answers on their own: connected clinicians and supporters in the health IT community who have put digital health into practice.

Dozens of interviews later, this book is the result. Chapters are taken from transcripts of the podcast and are edited only for clarity and length, used with the guests' support. My questions are in bold, followed by their responses. Preserving the conversational style of the audio interviews was key to making this a quick read. It follows a style similar to Gary Vaynerchuk's book *#AskGaryVee*, which is a collection of excerpts from his YouTube series.

Have I learned anything along the way? I'd like to think so. I have learned that physicians value their peers' opinions. I have learned that health system administrators, vendors and patient communities have a great deal of empathy for clinicians. But perhaps most importantly, I have learned that digital health can indeed improve patient care. It already is.

May you find this book useful as you read about some of the teams that are making it happen.

-I-
PARTNERING WITH PATIENTS

1
IT DOESN'T TAKE MORE TIME
A CONVERSATION WITH DR. DANNY SANDS

In this chapter, you will learn how to overcome the myth that engaging with patients takes more time. Dr. Danny Sands is a primary care physician, author, leading thinker in medical informatics and co-founder of the Society for Participatory Medicine. I invited him on the program after reading *Let Patients Help*, the revolutionary patient engagement guidebook he co-authored with "e-Patient Dave" deBronkart (see chapter 4). The book is inspiring because it is the real-life experience of a provider who improved a patient's life using technology and a new attitude.

When clinicians want to be engaged with their patients but aren't sure where to start, what do you tell them?

At one level, I teach them how to most effectively and engagingly use technology in the office. In other words, how to interact with the electronic health record and the patient at the same time.

It's a set of learnings that are critically important, especially now that physicians have to document everything in electronic health records.

It's important that physicians understand how to use this technology, how to listen to the patient and how to engage the patient in their record by sharing the information that's there, such as sharing the screen with them. That's a critically important piece.

But it goes beyond that. There is the whole attitudinal shift about sharing information beyond the visit. When you're talking about this, you're typically talking about patient portals. You should have a patient portal. I'm a big believer in transparency of all kinds, but particularly around what we're documenting in the patient's record, their test results and so on.

Coming back into the office, there's this phenomenon that physicians have when we are seeing patients and we're confronted with something where we're not sure what the answer is. It's an interesting dynamic because we're often taught that we need to know everything, but the reality is we can't know everything. When I talk to physicians in a non-threatening environment, I ask them, "How many of you think you know everything there is to know in your specialty?" And nobody raises their hand. Nobody.

Yet we are acculturated to believe that we must act like we know everything in front of colleagues, in front of nurses and in front of patients. So my learning in this area is admit to yourself that you don't know everything. Admit to your patients that you don't know everything. I call this "The Power of I Don't Know," which is when a patient asks you something and you don't know the answer. Don't have a deaf ear so that you pretend you didn't hear them and keep talking about something else. Don't walk out and ask one of your colleagues or look it up. Look them straight in the eye and say, "That's a really good question. I don't know. I don't know the answer to that."

I think it is shocking at first to some patients and it's uncomfortable for many physicians, but I think it's very, very important because it helps people understand that you can't know everything, and if you pretend you know everything, you're just lying.

Once physicians get comfortable saying, "I don't know," the next stage is saying, "I don't know" and following that up with, "Let's look it up together." Spend just a little bit of time getting at least the beginning of an answer with the patient right there on the computer. I think that's a very powerful thing to do.

The next set of early education would be to ask patients about their use of online health information. One of the most common things that people do online is look for health information. It's among the top three activities in every single demographic group. The problem is that many physicians either subtly or blatantly state that patients shouldn't read about health information online. More importantly, the patients shouldn't even be looking online. They think this is a terrible thing, and that the source of all knowledge should be from the physicians. That's not realistic because we know patients are going online looking for information. So we need to embrace that and understand that they're doing that.

My recommendation in this area is every year when you go through an annual review, you're asking patients about their smoking, their drinking, their drugs, their sexual habits and maybe strong religious convictions, and many of us even ask about whether they use any complementary alternative health techniques. A seminal national survey by David Eisenberg published in the *New England Journal of Medicine* in 1993 found that 1/3 of Americans were using complementary therapies but almost 3/4 never discussed it with their physicians. That's important. It's similar to going online to look for health information. Many people are using these techniques and not sharing it with their physicians because they feel like their physicians will be offended by this or not condone it.

So in a similar way, I ask every single one of my patients every time we do a wellness visit, "Do you go online? Have you gone online to look for health information? If so, what are some websites that you've found helpful?"

By the way, I write this down in their record. By having this conversation with patients, it helps them understand that you care where they're getting educated about their health. You care about that and you're receptive to it. By the way, this is also an opportunity to teach them. It rarely happens, but if the patient is getting their health information from an unscrupulous website or a highly biased website, that's an opportunity to have a conversation with them. It is opening the door to future conversations and leads them to future honest disclosures, which leads to the trusting, healing relationship that we need to have.

Finally, in the area of communication, many physicians are uncomfortable communicating with patients online. They feel like all communication should be in the office and if necessary, by phone. But we need to encourage patients to communicate with us online because it's more convenient for our patients and it's more convenient for us ultimately.

Physicians don't necessarily feel comfortable with that. They're afraid it's going to take up a lot of time or patients are going to be e-mailing them all the time and so on. In that situation, I say, "Look, just understand that there's not a large volume of work coming your way. That's been shown in study after study. And if you're uncomfortable with it, start by letting a handful of your most trusted patients use this technology, and then expand from there. Eventually, you're going to have all of your eligible patients using this. Any patient who's online will find this hugely satisfying and you're going to become increasingly comfortable with using it, as well."

A lot of clinicians still remain resistant to the idea that they should be empowering patients or using digital health tools. What are their pain points, and what do you say in response to those who remain skeptical?

The biggest thing I hear is that physicians are going to spend too much time: "I'm going to spend too much time, Danny. It sounds like an interesting idea, but I can't spend any more time. I'm already working late every day. I've got too much to do. I've got so many patients and so little time!"

So I think there is concern about the amount of time that all these activities take, which I think is a fundamental misunderstanding. To me, this is a change in attitude about transparency, about information sharing, about how we partner with patients, and how we make decisions. It's a change in attitude that does not have to obligate more time.

Here's a great example. We're talking about Open Notes, right? Physicians talk to patients. They spend their 15-minute visit with a patient and tell them things or they're discussing things and giving instructions. We agree on instructions. We know that as soon as patients leave the office, they remember less than half of what they were told. Every single physician I've ever spoken to in groups knows this statistic. They know this.

I ask them, "If you know that statistic, how many of you send your patients home with a video recording of your visits?" The physicians all sort of laugh nervously and say, "No, we don't." And I say, "Okay, then you probably just do an audio recording, right?"

And again, same nervous laughter. "No, we don't." And I say, "So you have to repeat yourself over and over and over and then you complain that your patients never remember anything that you tell them?"

That's fundamentally what we're talking about here. Patients can't remember everything that goes on in their visit and there's not enough time to write down a lot of what was said. So why not have that conversation—which is already essentially captured in your note—available to patients after the visit so they can check on that note and remember the plan that they discussed in the office? They can remind themselves by reading that note again and again, particularly before they come back for their next visit, so that you're achieving common goals and both have the same worksheet. That's powerful. That's an example of something that you can only do though this kind of transparency.

You recently blogged about a patient who was motivated to change his lifestyle simply by seeing his office notes about what you had documented about his visit. Why did it cause such a dramatic lifestyle change?

I had a patient whom we'll call "Joe," who came in for his annual visit. Joe was almost 60 years old. He came into the office for a checkup. Joe had not been taking care of himself for close to 20 years—as many years as I'd been taking care of him.

He had been overweight and was gaining more weight, not losing it. He never adopted any of the ideas and suggestions and encouragement that I gave him to change his lifestyle. Over the years, he got started on medicines that he took to reduce his blood pressure and cholesterol.

When he came to me for this particular visit, his weight had increased again. He was complaining of a number of symptoms. He was having back pain, a lot of heartburn and various other things. For each of these problems, I said, "I think if you were able to lose weight, it would really help you manage these things, but here's a medication that may help you."

He left the office with two or three new prescriptions and more encouragement to work on his weight. Because of his elevated blood pressure and various symptoms I asked him to return in a few months. When I walked into the office on the day of his scheduled visit, I didn't recognize him. There was Joe, wearing workout clothes, a muscle shirt and running shoes. I had never, ever seen him like this. I wasn't even sure I was in the right examination room.

I said, "Joe, what's going on?" He said, "Well, I was reading the note that you put online, and even though you wrote the note with me there and you talked about it openly all the time, I kept reading that word 'obesity.' I just sat and stared at that note online and decided I don't want to be that guy anymore. I signed up for a gym and got a Fitbit. I am now competing with 16 friends and family around the country. And with my Fitbit, I've found that I walked two million steps since I last saw you." It was just incredible. It's an incredible number of steps each day; I think 16,000 steps a day. He told me he lost weight; I could see by the numbers he'd lost well over 20 pounds.

He said all of his symptoms went away and he no longer needed medication to treat them. He made these dramatic changes through the combination of looking at his notes online and not liking what he saw there, but also through some self-motivation and social network motivation by using a Fitbit.

I think it's an important lesson that we should never give up and should always be transparent with people. If we think that the patient's obesity, for instance, is the cause of something, we shouldn't mince words. We need to be perfectly honest with our patients.

How does the health care community take participatory medicine to the next level?

I think there's a lot to be done in the areas of community. We need to convene conversations where we have patients and family caregivers face to face with physicians, developers, nurses and the whole spectrum of stakeholders to talk about how to solve the important problems facing health care. Together we can make health care better.

There are also things we can do in the area of advocacy to promote policy changes that will enable some of these technologies and tools. We need more research to document the effectiveness of these things. And finally, we need education.

Education is critical. On the one hand, we need health care professionals that welcome patients as collaborators in their health care. But we also need to educate patients, individuals and caregivers how to have more productive interactions with health care professionals. In fact, we should be educating people to be more engaged in their health and health care starting early in life— by the time they are confronted with a serious medical condition it's too late to change maladaptive behaviors, such as passivity.

Many people don't engage in earnest until they are confronted with a serious diagnosis, which is sometimes the trigger that can push them to participate in their own health and health care.

Joe was a great example that we talked about. He wasn't willing to engage no matter what I did with him until something tipped. There was some kind of trigger for him. But we need to encourage all patients and family caregivers to engage more in their health care.

I think all of these things are really important. We've got lots of work to do and we need all the help we can get.

2
SILENCE CAN BE CATASTROPHIC
A CONVERSATION WITH DR. FARRIS TIMIMI

In this chapter, you will learn why providers have a moral obligation to create and curate content for patients online, and how the absence of clinicians on social media can have catastrophic consequences. Dr. Farris Timimi is medical director for the Mayo Clinic Social Media Network. I invited Dr. Timimi on the broadcast because of Mayo Clinic's pioneering work in the field of social media under his clinical leadership. He has repeatedly shared how social media is not a substitute for clinical practice, which had been a longtime question in the medical community. Instead, we now have examples of how engaging on social media impacts the patient experience by offering unprecedented transparency. A great place to start is Mayo's social media accreditation course for health care professionals.

Mayo has partnered with HootSuite to create a social media accreditation program. Who is it for, and how does it help?

It's a tool that I've been very proud of. We worked very hard to create it. I think there's a growing recognition on the part of health care providers—including physicians, nurses and all allied health staff—that there are opportunities to use these tools correctly. But, like all tools, there are clear guidelines that need to be followed, clear orientation and clear training and onboarding that need to be incorporated.

Our intent in developing this social media accreditation was to assure that health care professionals at any realm or any level of a clinical practice could learn how to use these tools correctly. And it's just like any other tool in medicine. You certainly wouldn't give a number 11 blade, a scalpel, to a new trainee without providing them clear orientation, clear guidelines, clear, meaningful training, and testing how they learn. Our intent is to bring the same sort of academic rigor that we incorporate in every part of clinical practice to the aspect of social media in health care.

We've seen a dramatic uptick among health care professionals more than anyone else [the course is also offered to marketing and communications professionals]. Physicians, nurses and allied staff probably have been our largest user group because they're struggling right now. There's been a transition in the last four years in the conversations I have with health care professionals running social media. Initially, it was more an issue of how can I convince them this is important.

They now understand it's important. They clearly see the potential benefit, but they don't know how to use the tools, and, more importantly, don't know how to do so professionally, to do so in a fashion that brings respect and really maximizes the opportunity. So the majority of the people who have taken a course have been health care professionals, the frontline staff—physicians, nurses, nurse practitioners, mid-levels, the care providers we see as patients on a daily basis.

What's the biggest lesson you can share with health care professionals about using social media professionally versus personally?

I would highlight professionalism from a different perspective. I know what you're alluding to. You're alluding to the fundamental message that the power of social media is that the material created, the media we share, is archived and scalable. So it reaches beyond geography and beyond time, and that truly is the biggest fear health care professionals have. By professionalism, I mean the impact of our silence on clinical outcomes.

For example, if you look at vaccine compliance in the U.S. when the DP vaccine was introduced nearly 60-70 years ago, we saw a dramatic drop in the cases of whooping cough in the U.S. We went below 10,000 cases a year for nearly 37 years, but now we've seen an abrupt uptick in whooping cough cases that are approaching epidemic proportions in many states.

I believe our silence on issues like this, our inability to participate in the conversations online, has catastrophic outcomes in health care. And so by professionalism, I mean both the absence of unprofessional behavior, but also the presence of professional utilization of these tools, and it's both aspects that we focus on in our training.

How can a clinician use social media to impact the patient experience?

I think a patient's perspective of their health care trajectory is dramatically different from mine or from any other health care professional. The metrics or variables that are critical to me may not be the variables that are important to the patient. For example, my practice is heart failure. And, certainly, the variable that we often look at is how strong someone's heart is on an ultrasound study.

But what's really important to the patient is, "Can I do the things that I want to do on a daily basis and not get short of breath?" And that discrepancy in understanding can be challenging for both me and for the patients that I see. Part of the power of social is, frankly, as a listening strategy. Our patients are the lived experts of their disease trajectory. They've had the real-life experience of their individual diseases.

They can provide insight and understanding and comprehension that can be obtained in no other fashion from a large group in a matter of minutes in a one-hour chat. Moreover, issues that arise that impact outcomes can be learned, I believe, more readily and more feasibly from a broad, crowd-based strategy. We can gain early insight into potential issues that may arise running treatment modalities in a fashion that we could only obtain in the past through large clinical trials. So I think the capacity to tap into a patient's true experience can really be breathtaking.

The most prudent approach that I can think of is to join a Twitter chat. The patients have been predominant and have dominated this platform longer than we have. You can use a tool like Symplur to find the hashtags that are relevant—that's the health care hashtag repository, hashtags that are relevant to your particular disease practice that you're focused on.

Once you've identified those, you can use those hashtags to find Twitter chats or communities that gather online. And I would spend some time if I were a new provider to social media just lurking and listening. Let them know who you are. I was born in a small town in Tennessee. There's a small-town mentality to social. People are incredibly gracious. They're helpful. They'll guide you. They'll give you points and clues on how to use the tools correctly.

I think I would begin as a provider by listening. I also would begin as a provider, frankly, by looking at a course similar to ours before I began using these tools because you want to make sure that when you're online you realize you represent yourself, your practice, your profession, your enterprise, and the field of medicine that's relevant. So I would suggest new providers complete our course or course similar to that and then spend some time lurking and listening and letting patients know who you are and what you're there to do.

What are some advanced trends that you're seeing among the clinicians who have been on social media the longest?

I think they're beginning to recognize that social is not a replacement for clinical practice. That had been the hope, initially. There is still a profound value to the intimacy of a patient and a provider in the exam room together, but they're beginning to use and view these as additional tools. And they're thinking of clinical practice as morphing into two folds.

One is one-on-one. That means you as a physician in a room with a patient. The other is one-to-many, meaning you as a physician online with a community. And the tools have different metrics or variables that we examine. For example, I would think about social strategies for looking at community metrics for compliance, community metrics for health, community metrics for screening.

If you want to look at how many people in my community are being screened for high blood pressure, for diabetes, how can I improve those targets and those goals? How many kids in my community are wearing bike helmets? How can I improve those targets and goals? They're viewing social as a means to achieve those strategies. So they're beginning to see a bifurcation in practice with the power of an additional clinical tool that had never been there before.

How can providers use videocasting tools like Periscope and Facebook Live?

I think they're incredibly powerful tools. I think, frankly, we like watching videos. Not just we, but we on planet Earth. I think that's the only way you could defend or explain the incredibly high production numbers from YouTube, both hours viewed per month and hours produced per month. I think you can convey so much information in a video that can reassure, explain or engage a patient in a fashion that you can never achieve in writing and do so much more efficiently.

As you're well aware, Lee Aase did a Periscope video of his colonoscopy. I think the penetrance and reassurance people were able to see as a product of Lee beginning by live tweeting his preparation the night beforehand and then tweeting thereafter and then, frankly, seeing how quick the colonoscopy was, how rapidly they were able to complete the study. I've had patients who have told me, "I scheduled a colonoscopy because I saw your colleague's video online." That's a powerful message. If we could prevent one case of colon cancer, that's a profound yield on that investment.

Are there any other points about social media for clinicians that you'd like to convey?

I would reinforce the professionalism aspect. Again, by that, I don't mean the absence of unprofessional behavior. I think providers have a moral obligation to address health care literacy barriers, misperceptions and mistakes or misassumptions people make regarding their own health care. I think we do that very effectively in the clinical encounter, but I think the majority of providers are still exploring how to do so with a tool that's one-to-many like social media.

And I would, again, ask them to think carefully about how their silence on the social platform, where people not only spend significant time but also, as you're well aware, people have now evolved to the point that they view social media as a primary news source. They view Facebook's live feed or news feed as a primary source of news and information. Health care providers' silence in that platform can translate into other voices dominating the conversation.

There have been lots of studies conducted, for example, on YouTube videos on a variety of very specific diagnoses like high blood pressure, diabetes, rhinosinusitis or runny nose. And the majority of videos in many of those diagnoses focus on either misassumptions, alternative treatments that have not been proven, or product placement, people supporting and selling their own products.

It's because, frankly, providers are very reluctant to participate or produce content of value. Our capacity to either create or to curate content that's relevant to our patients on those platforms, producing media that is archived and scalable that can reach beyond time and geography, I think it's hard to argue against the argument that that is a moral obligation of health care providers in the digital era.

So I would really reinforce to the providers that are going to be listening that our silence on particular issues is catastrophic and lets other voices that have their own agenda dominate the conversation. And I would urge them to think carefully about the impact that has both on their clinical practice and on their community of relevance.

Where do you think that digital health is headed 3, 5 or 10 years from now?

I see a growing transparency in information access. In the prior era, the health care provider was the primary focus or source or owner of all the health care data and literature and guidelines that govern clinical care. Health care is growing at an astronomical rate. There's one new publication every minute produced in PubMed, which is a primary academic resource of relevance.

Our patients now have access to all that data, either through shared interactions through social platforms or in transparent data online. I believe we're approaching the point where our patients have the capacity to be both the lived experts of their disease but also to have meaningful insight into care decisions that can be powerful. And there's data to support this as well.

For example, look at what new diagnosis in the U.S. has the highest percentage of correct care being offered to that patient when they see the provider. The diagnosis that has the highest percentage of correct care being offered to the patient in the U.S. right now is breast cancer.

Because, in general, breast cancer patients are younger women who are electronically able, who are intelligent, who are online, who are going to social platforms where they're meeting with other patients who are also educated of their own volition, intelligent, articulate, and are telling them, "Before you see the provider, here are the five questions you need to ask the provider. Here are the decisions you need to make when you see a provider. When you choose a surgeon, this is what you need to think about before you pick a surgeon."

So I see this transparency being a powerful tool toward evolving to a patient partner that can join with us improving health care. I think our ability to improve outcomes by participating in that conversation, by walking with our patients through their disease to recovery, is profound. They're doing it right now in our absence, and when they do it correctly, it is a powerful outcome.

3
WE CAN'T KNOW ALL THE ANSWERS
A CONVERSATION WITH DR. WENDY SUE SWANSON

In this chapter, you will learn how ridiculous it is to think that any one person knows everything about all medical conditions and that patients know nothing. Dr. Wendy Sue Swanson, a.k.a. @SeattleMamaDoc, is a practicing pediatrician, blogger, author, speaker and executive director for digital health at Seattle Children's Hospital. I invited Dr. Swanson on the program because I am a huge fan of her proactive approach to communicating with patients and families. Because patients now use every resource at their disposal to research conditions and connect with care teams, she explains how digital health means more than just being on Facebook or using an EHR; it is being open-minded to partnering with patients and tech innovators.

How did you create a digital team at the hospital?

In 2013, I founded Digital Health, a department now consisting of five of us working to build and iterate new technology and bring new communications solutions into the hospitals. We are learning about how social media has changed information exchange and how patients and families search for health information. The majority of my time is now spent running a team working on these tools as well as the other roles that you described.

It's a work in progress. I think we've been successful in the sense that we partnered with an outside startup and engineers to build some new technology that we piloted within Seattle Children's Hospital. One is called Virtual Handshake, which you can read a little bit about at VirtualHandshake.org. It's a technology that we built to do the Google search for patients and families before they arrive in the clinic, and helps to reshape their interactions with providers.

When pediatricians or family docs refer patients with certain diagnoses to Seattle Children's Hospital, families are invited at the time of scheduling into a new community in the Virtual Handshake. Thus far, we have piloted this in our general surgery and gastroenterology departments. For example, say a patient family needs to see a surgeon under a diagnosis called inguinal hernia, a common abnormality that often baby boys are born with that needs surgical correction. They would then get invited into the Handshake. When they land there, it would say, "Hey Judy, we're excited to see you and baby Mark next Tuesday. Here's some information, videos, a map and handouts that the surgeon wants you to see even before you come."

This tool also allows families to invite other caregivers in a child's life to participate, so Dad, mother-in-law or a primary care doctor could all join. We also created a place for education at the time of discharge from the visit. What we try to do is say, "Can we be the physicians and researchers that we want to be before families come?" Then after they're done with their appointment, instead of handing them paper handouts, we could organize a link to the patient portal in addition to specific education handouts and our care plan all in one area. The primary caretaker could then invite anyone involved in their child's care to see this, not just those who are linked to the patient portal system. That's the pilot that we did over the last year or so. We've also done some other digitized education and peer-to-peer healthcare using an app called Tonic (see chapter 15).

What is your top tip for clinicians to engage in social media? What should they do, and what should they avoid?

First off, there are two reasons that most providers are not using social media. Number one is time, and number two is reimbursement. There's just no time and certainly no reimbursement for most physicians and care teams that are using social media. We do a couple of things when we join social media; we have a new tool to either narrowcast or broadcast what we know or what our opinions are, and we have another opportunity to hone our listening.

When I entered social media back in 2009, I was thinking kind of in a paternalistic way about health care. I wanted to detail through a mommy blog this story of new research, controversial parenting topics and ultimately vaccine science and safety, in a different way. The earnest, kind of gestalt, that's come over the years that I've now been doing it is that the tools are really profound listening devices. So I can hear when patients and families ask questions, and I can follow and build relationships with other like-minded thought leaders, reporters, parents and investigators across the country that help really inform me in an efficient way.

My top tip is to constrain yourself with a certain amount of time, say 10 minutes in the morning and 10 minutes at night, in a place where you want to be and where you feel energized, then think extremely strategically around what problem you want to solve. Maybe the problem is that I want people to really know how passionate I am about preventative health care, or I want people to know that we have a great resource in our community for smoking cessation, or I want families and patients to understand that I'm going to give them updates about our clinic flow when we have flu vaccine or when we don't, or I want families to understand that I really care about sleep and I'm going to curate links, information and ideas that resonate with me about sleep and they can follow me for that.

Don't frame it to yourself as, "I'm just going to go on social media because people tell me I need to do that to be 'relevant.'" Instead ask yourself, "Gosh, what do I care about, or where am I being misunderstood, or how do I want to build a footprint as a caregiver, care team, professional or expert?" This reframing to your passion creates your digital fingerprint. If you don't work for an organization that has good search engine optimization or a great bio, and if you don't have an otherwise easily packaged statement or purpose of work online, you can use these social tools as a way to reach your patients when they Google you as a provider.

Yes, there's this footprint of where we've been online, but you can also craft for the world who you are, what you do and what you're best at. I think that's where these tools can be profound. But by constraining them— using whatever tool you like—limiting it and using it to solve one singular problem can be a really great way for a clinician to just start tinkering around. My hunch is that you will start to feel a sense of connection, or an emboldened sense of personal purpose in what you're doing by sharing what you know in a social media tool like Twitter.

Are different types of information more engaging to your followers?

I think it kind of depends on who your followers are. On Twitter, I have a generous following that I'm very thankful for and with whom I interact regularly, around 30,000 people, and that group tends to be a lot of marketers, thought leaders, reporters, parents and other bloggers. I have private lists that I curate of pediatricians, family practitioners and other experts. In that space, what I share and how I listen is really focused on digital health and the role of physicians, patients and families, and peers in the health space, whereas my Seattle Mama Doc presence on Facebook is purely parenting information.

In social media platforms, I share blog posts that I write, funny posts and videos that come up that are relevant in the parenting space. I share personal anecdotes about my overwhelm with work-life balance or *New York Times* articles that I think resonate, so that's a different audience.

Then there's the LinkedIn/Doximity space and the traditional media spaces that I use really differently. I think not everybody is going to do what I do since my career has really evolved to be about how we communicate in health care both as patients and as providers. I like to help clinicians, researchers and business startups to utilize these tools. Find role models that you think do a great job and find people who do a really terrible job because those guardrails on both sides are really important.

For example: Twitter back in 2009 was a really intimate space in some ways in terms of the different groups who were working in health IT, but also physicians, care teams and hospitals working in social media. There were a bunch of disgruntled, burned-out physicians out there using pseudonyms or anonymous titles, ranting, but they were great guardrails for me to just watch and follow along. From them, I learned to ask myself, "When someone sends a message that makes me feel bad or that doesn't feel right, what does it teach me about how I can be a better leader?"

I love to encourage people also to diversify their audience. As a provider, you can't just follow health care people on Twitter. You have to follow celebrities, health care organizations and even neighbors. You have to learn how the tool is used universally so that you can help iterate, be relevant and take health care into a new place.

Why is it important to engage with patients' families?

Pediatricians and family practitioners are always caring for two sets of people in every visit: the patient for whom they're advocating, and the family who are the stakeholders in those decisions. Loved ones who also tend to suffer or feel vulnerable in times of stress and illness.

I started out by writing a parenting blog. I'm typically writing for family members and caregivers. The other reason that I think so much about family is that one of our most untapped resources in the health space is the expert patients and the caregivers who help support them during times of illness.

We haven't really brokered a great place for caretakers in health care, so part of my role in building that minimal viable product of Virtual Handshake was really to say a couple of things: Let's get care teams or providers—social workers, nurses, nurse coordinators, doctors and surgeons—involved in using digital tools to deliver what they know. And let's also have an organization acknowledge how important it is not just to care for and communicate with the person who's at the bedside with the patient, but ultimately the other people in a child's life that might benefit from having the education to help support a child, continue a care plan or understand more about what's going on. Through another endeavor, we created digitized education for families after liver transplantation. We teach them about the medicines their child is taking, how and why immunosuppressives work and what to do. In every chapter where we're providing education on medicines, lab draws and immunosuppression, we have content that's been co-created by patients and families as well.

Instead of just saying, "Here's the kind of paternalistic way that we're going to tell you what to do," we're also going to tee up families who have had a liver transplant before and leverage their wisdom, expertise and experience right alongside the clinicians to broker more meaningful relationships. Those who have been down that road before you have a lot to share, not just because of empathy, but because of their wisdom and their resources.

Seventy percent of parents are going online and doing so-called "sharenting." They're asking their crowd on Facebook about the rash that their kids have, or if they should be getting vaccines. They're thinking about where they're going to get health care. Are they going to go to Minute Clinic? Target? Walgreens? The regular pediatrician's office? Or are they going to go to the big hospital?

We have to remain relevant by helping understand who the influencers are right now for patients and families. Doctors will always be, I think, the most trusted resource in a time of stress, pain, agony or suffering. I think we have to help broker these new relationships.

As a clinician, does it offend you when patients research their own conditions or do you incorporate their questions and empower them?

It doesn't make any sense that we wouldn't want patients and families to be doing research. It's archaic to think that we as providers would hold all of the answers in a time of personalized and precision medicine. The era is coming where patients and families can hack into their own resources, learn from each other and sequence their genome. I think if we can't tolerate a Google search before someone comes in, we're rendering ourselves mute.

There was a meme recently with an image of a coffee mug that said something like, "Your Google search is not the equivalent of my MD." I remember seeing this and thinking, "Really? Is that really your belief? You can know more about some aspects of health care than anyone in the world and yet your patient might bring something to you that you didn't know about."

In the beginning of my practice in medicine, which was almost 10 years ago now, I remember patients and families bringing me things about vaccines and I'd say, "Oh, I don't know," and then I'd Google it with them, find a resource and realize that they had something they were teaching me. Whether it was about aluminum, or fetal parts being used in the production years ago in vaccine development, or whatever their worry was—they were helping actually provide an education for me. It's my responsibility to go find a source that I trust, understand the science and explain it. But I think we can't provide health care the way that we always used to, and hold all of the advice ourselves and not open up to let families resource information in different ways. It's just too expensive and laborious to do it that way.

For me, building new tools was really just about acknowledging that the role of health care, hospitals, some specialists and primary care doctors in the future is earnestly going to be the art of great, personalized curation. You can imagine a world where a patient says, "Okay. Here's my genome." It's something like a 23andMe but institutionalized, where they get their genome sequence, they find out what their risks are and then an organization says, "Gosh, based on this profile, here's the information that our experts recommend that you read before your 40-year-old visit, before your 45-year-old visit, what we think you should read at 60 and gosh, you just had a new baby. Here's the information we want you to have at 10 days of life. Here's the information we want you to have before your 6-month visit."

How much better is that than trying to pack it all into a 15-minute visit when it's not personalized or not based on filters, diagnostics and predictability? Patients will do their research and then it's our job to be there with them asynchronously, virtually and in person and be relevant by being a really smart curator. You go to the MoMA in New York because a curator decided what they thought was most interesting and valuable in modern art. We want to go to a doctor who's well-trained and who knows what's most important, and also most helpful when people are making decisions about both their prevention and their illness. I'm intolerant of thinking that families shouldn't be involved and guiding us in ways of what's important to them.

What is the #1 piece of advice that you're sharing with patients and sharing with families right now?

I'd say it is to trust your instincts. Use every resource you have, whether it be your crowd, the Internet, or the specialized health centers in your region. Utilize both the expert, conglomerate aggregated care centers around the country and your communities online. Use your peer networks. Go online and find as much as you can and then be as squeaky as you need to be to get the best health care you can. I want people to feel that they have a really big role in their health and it's very hard to feel that way in a system that isn't yet designed to empower them.

There are clinicians all over who value and involve families and patients beautifully, but our health systems are lagging a bit because we want to be so safe. We want to provide valuable care under the guidance of the organizations that supervise the safety of hospitals. But it isn't yet totally prioritizing the role of patients and families speaking up in a participatory way. We're making strides, but people should use every tool they possibly can to get the best care for themselves, and the best preventative efforts for themselves and their families.

4
PARTNER WITH PATIENTS
A CONVERSATION WITH "E-PATIENT DAVE" DEBRONKART

In this chapter, you will learn why understanding the voice of the patient is crucial to improving care and patient satisfaction. "e-Patient Dave" deBronkart is a leading spokesman for the patient engagement movement. I invited Dave on the program because few have ever been able to match his articulate perspective of the relationship between patient and provider. Between blogging, social media, keynote speeches around the world and co-authoring the patient engagement handbook *Let Patients Help*, his influence drives change in all aspects of health care. His TED Talk entitled "Let Patients Help" for years was in the top half of the most-watched TED Talks of all time. Dave is a survivor of metastasized kidney cancer that was almost sure to be fatal. But he frequently credits the empowering relationship of his primary care physician doctor, Dr. Danny Sands, with helping him kick cancer to the curb.

How have attitudes changed towards patient engagement in the clinician community since you first started advocating for it?

It's important to realize, after several years of talking about patient engagement and patient empowerment, that our conception of what empowerment and engagement are continues evolving, and that this is a time of great culture change. Sometimes it seems we are approaching a culture war in this area (not that a war is necessary).

But as in any social movement where people's conception is evolving, there are a lot of people who say, "Oh, great. New things are possible," but there are always some people who say, "No. This is wrong. It's not true." Some people say, "It's offensive to me," and they resist and fight back.

Like all change attitudes—the women's movement, race relations, etc.—at first there's skepticism because people have never seen the new world as possible. Then people start to realize it's possible, and we start moving forward.

We now have a clearer picture of what is possible when patient engagement and empowerment are done right. Now we face the question, so how the heck do you make it work? That's where we're learning. Five years ago, I gave two different talks in the same year, and in both cases an experienced older doctor came up to me and said, "Crap. My patients can't do any of this stuff."

I just wonder to what extent that is self-fulfilling: if he believes it's not possible, it would make no sense to even try, right?

These days, I don't hear the same things. The trade press is much more filled with questions, conferences and speeches about how to actually do patient engagement and empowerment.

At the same time, I gave a talk in London last year where I

said, "Inevitably. The empire strikes back." I've never seen a clearer example of that than in Belgium. A key part of patient engagement and empowerment is welcoming the work when a patient tries to educate themselves by getting information online. A lot of people say, "Watch out. There's garbage on the Internet," and that's certainly true. But who doesn't know that?

Some patients think that if it's on the Internet it must be true. I would say those people are naive. But on the other hand, it clearly is possible for patients to find useful information.

Here are two contrasting stories from overseas to illustrate the point. The Belgian government, starting in late 2014, starting running a Google ad campaign, where in Belgium if you Google a symptom the top search result that comes back is paid for by the Belgian government and says, "Don't Google it." It leads to a professional, ad agency-produced video that shows a couple at home. It starts out where the husband's got a boo-boo on his finger and the wife bandages it, and then she goes online.

Like a babbling idiot, within 90 seconds they've convinced themselves he's dying from bleeding warts on his head. The commercial ends with "Don't Google it. Consult a professional." When I blogged about this a couple months ago, I said, "Who says those two things are mutually exclusive. Why not Google it *and* consult a professional?"

The indictment of that Belgian government policy is a story that came out last summer, where a few years ago in the United Kingdom, a 19-year-old who had been cured of liver cancer started to not feel well again. She and her mother were educating themselves on the Internet, and they found a patient group and some information saying, "Guess what? This does come back sometimes." The doctors said, "Stop Googling," and she died. So this year, those doctors in the NHS, the English National Health

Service, apologized for their role in her death.

Now, I'm not saying those doctors were arrogant jerks. I have no idea who they are. It's just that the world has changed since they were trained. A generation ago, it was ludicrous to think that a young patient and her mother at home would find information that professional physicians did not know. But that's no longer ludicrous; it's *real*.

Once you accept that something might be possible and useful, the next question is often, "All right. How do I do it?" I saw that when the health policy journal *Health Affairs* came out with their entire theme issue on patient engagement in February of 2013. Without even realizing it, they had multiple implied definitions of patient engagement throughout the different articles. The editors didn't even notice the differences.

Some people, when they talked about patient engagement, were only talking about getting patients to do what they're told. The most egregious example was that article from Pharma, where their belief seemed to be that patient engagement was getting people to buy the prescription. There was no capacity anywhere in that article for the idea that maybe a thinking patient would say either, "Well, I don't want that," or "I want it, but frankly it's not worth the amount of money you guys are charging. I'd rather tough it out."

They said that they have given up on patient engagement, and they meant that patient engagement was a way to get people to do what they're told and basically give the amount of money to the prescription that they were instructed to give.

Now, there are a decreasing number, but some clinicians will say, "No. I'm the one with the medical degree. I'll ask the questions." In which case, you the patient may decide to suck it up, or you may decide to look for another one. But then, from the physician side, I asked my primary physician Danny Sands, who is one of the co-founders of the Society for Participatory Medicine, what his advice to clinicians is.

He's pretty well-known in the field of informatics, medical records, technology. Here is a doctor who clearly is not a hyper-radical hippie wacko, who has been doing this successfully for 15 years. The reason physicians like his advice is because they know it's not coming from somebody who hasn't walked in their shoes.

I hope now that if we can envision the patient as an active partner, with every right to have their hands on data, that we will start implementing that as a reality. I hope everyone is aware of the now famous OpenNotes Movement. It's not a software product. It's just the idea that your hospital, your provider's office sort of drills a hole through the patient portal, so you too can now see the so-called "visit notes" that clinicians write to each other.

Most patient portals are clinically useless, except for looking up lab results. They'll let you see what your blood tests were. But you can't get in and see what the doctors and nurses wrote to each other about you. Well, with OpenNotes, they just kind of drill a little hole through there and let you see what the doctors and nurses wrote to each other. Amazingly, if you just Google "OpenNotes" all the evidence says good things happen when patients are informed.

How do Meaningful Use requirements impact patient engagement?

Time will tell. The fact that a mandate comes out of Washington doesn't mean that people actually do it. Everybody talks about HIPAA in terms of privacy violations. Well, HIPAA also says that you have a right to every word that people have written about you. They're allowed to charge certain amounts, but they are not allowed to say no.

Believe it or not, HIPAA is administered within HHS, Health and Human Services, by the Office for *Civil Rights*. It is a federal civil rights violation for somebody to not give you your records, and yet hardly anything has been done to enforce that. I always talk about what's newly possible and how if we don't do those things we'll never achieve what's fully possible. I'm hoping that people will see this can be a good thing and help move forward.

You and I own our own financial data. We collect it from various places in Quicken or Mint.com, and we can authorize a tax accountant or financial advisor to look at it; not only look at it, but edit it and work in it.

Aside from the fact that there are no controls to make sure only accurate data gets into the record, for the most part, these systems do not talk to each other yet. There's a move toward interoperability, but it'll be years before it's a reality everywhere.

In the meantime, nobody in health care is guaranteed to be talking to others to make sure everyone has the latest information. It is up to you, the patient or family member, to collect the information and be sure that the next doctor or nurse that you talk to is aware of it. It's very common for one system to say something different from what another system says.

I'll give you a simple example that nearly killed my mother a few years ago, and this is so trivial and yet it's so perfect and so dangerous. She was discharged from the hospital after having a successful hip replacement and transferred to a rehab place to get her physical therapy and post-op treatment. Somehow, her thyroid condition came across backwards: she's hyper, and the note somehow said hypo. So the best doctor in the world at the rehab place could've prescribed the opposite medicine from what she needed, and real harm could have happened to my mom because of a simple, stupid, dangerous data error. Not okay!

Is there anything else you'd like to share about patient engagement?

Well, first of all, for heaven's sake, do OpenNotes. If the people you work with are not familiar with it and don't realize how it's a no-brainer, just Google "OpenNotes" and you'll get all the literature, stories, statistics and publicity. Please do that.

Think about yourself, really, with your child, your spouse, or your elderly parent, in crisis, and the sense that you have of, "Is there anything I can do to help?" There is a lot more you can do to help if you're allowed to look at the data.

It is culture change. You may get push-back. But cultures evolve when a majority of people say, "This is the right way to do things."

Finally, be aware that gadget data (like fitness wristbands) is turning out to be truly useful. Gadget data is over-hyped at present, but that always happens when new things come along, It doesn't mean that everything that comes in will be solid gold.

I'm a skeptic about whether so-called Big Data will ever actually produce great value. But I will tell you right now, I have two different fitness wristbands on my wrist, just because I want to compare them. One I got for free, and the other one I bought. They count steps differently. They have different features. I hate parts of both of them. During my successful weight loss campaign I used MyFitnessPal for tracking food, and my Wi-Fi bathroom scale and Runkeeper for tracking my activities.

In four months I lost 30 pounds, and became someone who gets uncomfortable if I don't get out to walk, and sometimes run a bit. A year later a near miracle happened: I did become an actual runner, and lost another ten pounds.

And it's not just me. My doctor has another patient who has just been overweight, clinically obese for years, and he started using a Fitbit and he has lost 30 pounds. When Dr. Sands talks about it, it's hard to believe.

And here's the deliciously ironic thing: Dr. Sands can't see all my device data in his big, fancy computer. You see how ironic that is? People say, "Patients won't get off their butt and do the work, and it causes all kinds of problems and diabetes." Well, what happens when I start having this cloud of data around me that he can't see? That's why Eric Topol, the famous cardiologist, published a book a little bit more than a year ago called *The Patient Will See You Now*, because we're beginning to have this world of home device data. When every other industry is computerized and starts using emerging technology, quality goes up, prices go down and consumers get more power. The same is happening with health care.

5
YOU CAN'T COMPLAIN ABOUT BAD CONTENT IF YOU AREN'T CREATING GOOD CONTENT
A CONVERSATION WITH DR. JUSTIN SMITH

In this chapter, you will learn how to counter bad health information on the Internet by publishing good information instead. Dr. Justin Smith, better known as @TheDocSmitty, is a practicing pediatrician, blogger, podcaster and medical advisor for digital health for Cook Children's Hospital. I invited Dr. Smith on the program because he advocates the value of clinicians being active with social media and engaging patients. Years ago, he chose not to complain about patients who empowered themselves and instead gained institutional support to build a national name for himself—and consequently for his hospital.

What are some of the latest topics that you've been talking about on social media?

I stay pretty active on two different channels. I'm active on Facebook and Twitter as The Doc Smitty and I find that both of them are good places to interact with various people. I do find that the audiences are quite different. I have quite a few patients who follow me on Twitter, not direct patients, necessarily, but people with children from our local area and even nationally. And then I find on Twitter that I have much more of a professional following with other doctors and media folks and reporters, people who are interested in what we are having to say.

Looking back through what we've covered recently, I do write my own blogs and those we've covered, for instance, why we haven't seen a lot of flu in our area to this point. As far as more news topics, we've covered the Zika virus which is something that we saw as kind of a trend of people having concerns about, so we addressed that. Then we also try to cover evergreen topics that are just general pediatric topics that our audience would also be interested in.

How do you know when a topic will generate that type of response, and how do you know it's something that's okay to talk about?

We have a list of topics in pediatrics that are particularly hot right now. Vaccines are always going to be a big one and so we know when those go out. I ask my editor not to release those on a day that I'm off work. So, I want to be around so that I'm listening to the conversation and able to be engaged.

We have other topics that we've covered such as essential oils, use of chiropractors in pediatrics, and we just kind of know what those topics are that are particularly hot. Also news items that potentially present a danger to our patient population that we know can be really interactive and really need us to be involved in engaging the conversations.

So, we have our list of concerns and then you never know; sometimes things surprise you. You'll put some things you think are relatively benign and end up getting a pretty good response, both positive and negative.

What's the value to you as a clinician to be out there spending that much time on social media?

It's really valuable to me as far as learning about what my parents who are in my office are concerned about. But then also I really feel that we are getting to a point now where people are getting so much information online. Every time I see a new study come out, it seems like the percentage of people who have searched for their health conditions online gets higher and higher and I really feel like it's almost becoming, at least for some of us, a duty to be out there and providing good information.

That's really why I got into it from the beginning. There was all this talking and condescension about the patient who brings in a lot of information they got online and I finally got to a point where I said, "If we're not really creating good information, how can we complain about the bad information they're bringing in?" I think it's important that we are out there creating and sharing good data and good information if we want our patients to have access to it.

One of the things we always teach about social media is that you should listen first. I think through my time with social media, and I've really tuned my ears into what patients are thinking, what they need and what they would like for a pediatric experience.

Communication with pediatricians is, in a lot of ways, dated. I still hear people who have to call in and leave a message when they have a question, and they might not get a call back for several hours. How can we possibly let that happen when there are so many tools that could facilitate communication between parents and their pediatrician? So that was really the first bucket that we wanted to go after.

Another one was medical decision-making in pediatrics. Even asking, "What type of visit do you need?" was completely paternalistic, and we're basically saying, "Oh, we don't think you're competent enough to tell us how you should get in touch with us," or, "We need you to come and deal with this problem," that probably we just need a phone call. Maybe even a little text message would be plenty to address the issue.

And yet we're saying, "No, no, no, you're going to have to come in for this." And partly there's a payment issue there, and there are other barriers that made that the case. But I feel like if you do the right thing for the families and they tell someone else and you get a new check-up in the place of that ill visit that you handled online, well, then the payoff is even better.

I think the last bucket I would say where we needed a big change was just inefficiency of visits and how people would come in. Basically, they answered the same questions multiple times. They leave frustrated because the time that they did have with the doctor, they didn't actually feel like the doctor was present. So I think that's another area where we can just streamline the process, make it to where parents can get as much of that work done as they can before they come in, do most of it when they're not in front of the staff or the doctor.

When I come in, it's not focused on this basic level of what

I tell every two-month-old checkup. They've already got all that. Well, it's what's next and what's next-level and what can they take home that's very personalized for them that answers their question, not just what I thought was important.

How have you gained support with hospital administration?

I came to Cook Children's about two and a half years ago and at that point, I was already doing some Facebook and blogging on my own. I had a little bit of a voice already built out in my little sphere, which was a small town in West Texas. But as I came over here, they were actually in a process of transitioning over to a newsroom-style publication and moving away from a twice-a-week blog to actually creating news in the pediatric space for our area, for our state, and really for the country.

And it was really fortuitous that I came along when that ball had already started rolling. I was able to come onboard and say, "Hey, I'm willing to oversee this. You can be sure that we're providing good information." Then I helped to recruit other physicians to contribute as well. We have a great team that has interacted well with our clinical staff for years but just having a doctor on the team, I think lends us some credibility that increased our participation from clinicians across the system.

Is there still some give and take? Do some administrators still wonder why you are spending so much time on digital health?

Yeah, I think there are probably some who understand the value more than others. But overall, they're just very supportive and they've seen the traction that we've gained and the reach that we have, the level of connection and engagement that we have with our followers. And once they see that, certainly they're much more open to trying new and different things with us.

What statistics do you use to measure success?

As a digital marketing team, we are looking at statistics past reach. But still when you're communicating with people who don't understand that, sometimes reach is a really powerful discussion point. And it's something that's fairly easy measurable over time and it can be something that they understand. We particularly are more interested in engagement on our team. We think that's an important measurement for us.

Do you use any mobile health tools in patient care, and why do you like them?

We're looking at integrating more digital health tools and mobile health tools into the pediatric clinic. I think there is a lot of momentum and movement in digital health, so we're not alone.

One of the things that we're seeing a bit of a gap in is through the day-to-day digital health tools that help the healthy family, the healthy child, who's needing checkups and routine care to help make their life easier. As we prepare to open a new clinic, we focused on building it out in a way that the technology is patient friendly and not an interference in our relationship with them.

Tools like telemedicine and remote ear exams are some of the things that we plan to have the day we roll out. We've done pilots and studies and feel comfortable with those two technologies as early technologies we want to adopt, basically to make things more efficient for our families so the things that we can handle remotely without a trip in, we can do. But then still providing solid pediatric care in office. So, it's not a replacement for good pediatric care, but it could be a supplement.

As a clinician, what do you do to empower the families of the patient during their care?

In pediatrics, we're pretty fortunate. A lot of the things that we treat and take care of are self-resolving issues and the kids generally are going to do well and get healthy. And then there are also parents who ask us parenting questions, things from your experience, what-have-you-seen type situations.

Also, I think we are getting better about giving parents the options for different ways to receive care. And I think that asking them what they would like early on is important because if you get down the path of some treatment option and realize that it wasn't their goal from the very beginning, it's hard to back track.

Yeah, I think that's the direction health care is going. Parents are getting so much noise parents from all different channels and patients. Strategically, we're not competing against just other health care providers, we're operating in the same space that big industries with huge marketing budgets are working in. We have to be clever about how we get that messaging out there and use tools that could affect change.

What's the advantage of having technology in the waiting room?

We're trying to deliver as much as we can, even ahead of time, before they get into the waiting room. The waiting room is the fallback option to not seeing the form or not getting it done ahead of time before they come into the visit. So our goal is to have them walk in, be completely registered and have a big chunk of their clinical history taken before they walk in the door.

But with their input, with the ideas I had, we built the waiting room teeny tiny and more extra rooms, because we want patients to walk in ready to go, and, "Oh, hey. You're ready to be seen. You can go on back to room 6," and there may just be a slight little pause at the front desk to let them know where to go, and not spend a lot of time out in the waiting room filling out forms.

And that goes back towards this patient design idea. We tried to do it, and I think it's a buzzword right now, and unfortunately that means its going to start to lose its meaning to some degree. Everybody will think they're supposed to be doing it, so they say they are.

Some people say, "Oh yeah, we're in social media," but they're just broadcasting their press releases over and over again. It's the same thing with patient-centered design, I think. It's getting to the point where we need a term that means "real patient-centered design" and not "because I know I'm supposed to do it."

I think you take small successes, and then you try to replicate those and make them grow over time. That's what we've seen, is like, "Oh well, okay, so they were on board with telemedicine, well, let's try bringing this on. Would you guys think that would be a good idea?" and then if they unanimously say yes, well then it's easy to know that that's the next direction to go.

It's interesting you talk about user experience. When you're building a website, it's the same concept as how is the user going to walk through this information? How are you going to get them from point A to point B to point C as easily and efficiently as possible?

So user experience is a huge piece of the digital experience, but the idea that you're taking it from "How does it work on a website or a tablet or an app?" to "How do they walk through the office? What are their biggest issues?" Yeah, who wants to take a kid with a fever or feeling crappy out of the car to then sit someplace and ask them to be quiet when they're already asleep in the car, and oh, the room's ready, I can go right in? I'm sorry, it's brilliant, well done, you.

Another thing is telemedicine, I'll have plenty of parents who never use it, and that's fine. But I want them to have the choice to use it should the need arise. And if you're not providing the choice, but just complaining that they're going to urgent care, I just don't like hearing people complain when they're not providing an equivalent or good service.

And so, there's social media, after-hours care and telemedicine. We can't continue to complain about these companies that are doing it and seeing our patients do telemedicine if we're doing nothing to provide even 75% of that service. Maybe we don't have the same hours as they do, but at least we give them that as an option. Well, if we're not doing anything, what are we complaining about?

6
PATIENT SATISFACTION SCORES AFFECT REIMBURSEMENT RATES
A CONVERSATION WITH MANDI BISHOP

In this chapter, you will learn the correlation between digital engagement, patient satisfaction scores and reimbursement rates. Mandi Bishop was named #1 on the 2016 #HIT100, recognizing her as the top social media influencer in health IT. She was also named to HealthData Management's list of the Most Powerful Women in Health Care IT. I invited her because she has a deep understanding of—and empathy for—both clinicians and patients.

How do you get clinicians to overcome their pain points about empowering patients and adopting digital health?

The carrot-and-stick approach is right, and I struggle with this quite a bit. From a carrot perspective I'm always trying to bring it back to the language that is universally understood for corporate America, and that's whether you're an independent physician practitioner or whether you're a very large hospital system, your HCAHPS scores talk.

At the end of the day, your reimbursement rate from CMS matters and so having a positive impact on patient experience is something that is actually quantifiable and is now being measured and refined on a continual basis. Physicians and hospital systems have a vested interest in meeting their patients where their patients live, and their patients are increasingly living on social media.

I think that the latest research from Pew indicates that more than 40% of all the adult population in the U.S., everyone 18 and up, across all income levels, all race and ethnicities, are on a social media network daily. And I think that the number has reached over 70% of them who are accessing all of these networks via their smart phone. So we live in an app-powered society and social engagement is how our members and patients interact with each other.

I think about my daughter. I think about her growing up and her friends—Millennials—don't talk to each other anymore. They text. And so if you don't show me something on a screen, it doesn't exist, and the more that health care providers understand how a lack of engagement in a digital context is going to negatively impact their reimbursement rates when it comes to scores, the more they understand that direct correlation between digital engagement and patient satisfaction, patient experience scores, the better it is that they will, if they have been reluctant, at least they will be willing to try.

I hate to have to have that conversation. There are certainly lots of health care providers who are excited about the opportunity to go digital. They want omni-channel communications with their patients, but there are obviously budgetary constraints that you have to understand and you have to be able to help those providers take tiptoe steps into the digital realm because there are things that are not required. They have to do Meaningful Use if they are part of the CMS program. Now they're going to have to comply with MACRA.

If their organization is on the value-based care APAP program, they're part of an ACO, so there are all these other mandates that are absolutely required that they have to be able to allocate their time and dollars to before they're able to pay attention to digital communication strategies. And I think that's a business imperative that a lot of us who are very excited about omni-channel communications miss. We know that it is something that matters. We know that it's something that can truly transform patient relationships but we fail to consider all of the other pressures that the providers are under and having to meet.

So showing clinicians how to do very low-cost, entry-point digital communications with their patients is key. Social media is a great one. It's free. Getting a Facebook account is free. Setting up a Facebook page is free. Setting up a Twitter account is free. Instagram is free. These are all ways that you can at least begin to engage. You can at least dip your toe in the water and even if you don't post anything, you can at least start to listen and understand how your patients engage.

And it also develops kind of a more personal one-on-one relationship that so many of us are lacking with our doctors right now. We talk about customer loyalty and wanting to keep our patient panel. We want to be able to reduce the churn rate.

So part of the way to do that is to at least establish a digital presence and start to make that presence known to your patients, even if you have to start dipping your toe in the water with freely available platforms and taking more of a listening approach than a high-touch engagement.

What is the initiative to involve more patients at industry conferences, and why do we need it?

It's funny because the first several years that I went to HIMSS, I was just so excited to be there and so awed by the size and scope of HIMSS that it did not occur to me that we were all talking about engaging with patients, but I didn't hear any patients. The closest I came to hearing patients and seeing the patient presence at HIMSS was Regina Holliday who is just a wonderful, amazing patient advocate.

For anyone who does not know, look up #thewalkinggallery and @ReginaHolliday on Twitter. Regina has become an accidental patient advocate and an open data advocate because of an experience that she had losing her husband. Anyway, she was a very vibrant, vital presence at HIMSS, but I was so stoked to be there and I'm so lost in my own geeky world that I didn't realize that patients weren't there, let alone there in mass.

And then I became close friends with Casey Quinlan (@Mightycasey) and a group of other patient advocates, Jan Oldenburg and Kate Rowe and Carly Medosch and Jess Jacobs. I mean the list goes on. But they started to open my eyes to their lack of a voice or their perception of a lack of a voice, not just at the conference itself but in the planning of the conference and being able to get their talks accepted into the conference.

They're not just helping plan the events for the inclusion of patients but helping plan the educational sessions that the patients were included and appreciated at the same level as the industry experts. And the folks of the Society for Participatory Medicine, the founding members Dr. Danny Sands, "e-patient Dave" deBronkart, really opened my eyes to the need for a best practice of inclusion at HIMSS, and a gentleman by the name of Lucien

Engelen came up with a patients included charter.

It's #PatientsIncluded and if you go to patientsincluded.org it talks about five charter clauses for including patients at conferences, things like making sure that there are appropriate ADA facilities for patients, making sure the patient track is included from an educational standpoint.

We talked about how to help HIMSS meet the charter clauses of the Patients Included movement, and then how to go beyond that and get the sponsoring organizations—the exhibitors at HIMSS—to really buy into the Patients Included concept and start funding a consortium so that patients can be included at more events. Not just included but assisted to get there.

The hardest part isn't the brainstorming. It isn't coming up with all the ways to make this a win-win proposition. Those are the relatively easy pieces. The hard piece is mobilizing and organizing this massive people who want to be engaged because unfortunately, whether we're patients or whether we're just advocating on behalf of this Patients Inclusion program, we're all volunteers.

Funding is also a problem. We all want to do good but there are finite amounts of time and finite amounts of money.

7
CREATE HIGHLY ENGAGED PATIENTS AND FAMILIES
A CONVERSATION WITH DR. TANYA ALTMANN

In this chapter, you will learn why you should think about the patient's family. Dr. Tanya Altmann is a bestselling author, television parenting expert and practicing pediatrician. I invited her on the program because she has a national TV audience and incorporates social media outreach into her daily routine, all while seeing patients and raising three active boys. She puts highly engaged patient care at the center of her concierge practice by making connected health tools work for her in her everyday workflow. She gives a blueprint for using an array of tools from remote ear exams to Facebook to patient email alerts on her Apple Watch. The result is creating highly engaged patients and families without sacrificing time, one of our most valuable assets.

What is your top tip for clinicians to engage in social media? What should they do, and what should they avoid?

That's a highly debated topic. I think if you talk to a variety of physicians, everyone will give you different advice and they'll all have great advice and tips and some of it is just learning from our own experience because this is a whole new world.

We're all learning how to navigate the world of social media, especially when it comes to our patients and families in our office. So with my families in my office, I do use email. I put it directly into the EHR (electronic health record); that way they can email me whenever they have any questions.

Often depending on the topic, I might write back them to them and say, "I'm going to call you in five minutes" because I feel that in many cases I can't be face to face, but a voice to voice conversation over the phone or Skype is really needed. I don't want to lose anything in translation when we're just typing words back and forth.

I also use Facebook and Twitter for my practice as well as my Dr. Tanya, which is a little more of a national profile. Really with social media, I just try to share important health information for families. So it could be something like the new LEAP study that came out on the importance of getting peanut products early in a baby's diet to help decrease the risk of peanut allergy later in life. It could be information on the new Zika virus going around or when we had the measles outbreak here in southern California.

It's really more general information and I try not to give direct patient advice via social media. But often people will write in and ask questions and I will try to answer it in more general terms to help teach more of my audience. Then often I will recommend that they reach out to their own pediatrician.

Are you recommending a mix of the communication element of social media but also acknowledging that's not the place to provide medical advice?

Exactly. I think it's a slippery slope. Someone might tweet and say, "Hey, my toddler doesn't like to eat vegetables. What do you recommend?" Then I would say in general when I have picky toddlers, this is how I recommend getting them to eat a wide variety of vegetables, plant a garden, go grocery shopping, things like that.

If their tweet was, "My toddler has a 103 degree fever and a cough. Is this the flu?" I might give a sentence on flu but then I will say, "Please see your own pediatrician or if your toddler has a fever over 104, a fever for more than three days, has trouble breathing or looks sick, make sure you see your own doctor."

So you always want to cover yourself and make sure you're giving the right advice so no one misreads it and doesn't seek medical treatment when they might need it.

You mentioned using email and tying in with the EHR. Does that replace a patient portal for you as your primary means of communicating with patients?

You know, it really does. I love my EHR. It's a pediatric-specific EHR and I would love to use the patient portal more. However, it doesn't have the ability to alert me through the patient portal. So therefore if somebody sends an email, it might sit there unless it's during business hours or my laptop is open.

So what I do—and different experts have given me different opinions on this—I have a special email that I use for my patients. And I send it directly to the EHR, and I make sure that everything is followed up on.

When I get that email, it alerts me on my Apple Watch. I have my Apple Watch set to only vibrate for patient emails. That way I can read and respond right way. For me, that's actually one of the ways that my families prefer to communicate with me and that I prefer to get alerted whether it's nighttime, weekends, I'm on vacation during the day, just with a little tap on my wrist.

All patients know the instructions and what they can email me, what they can't, if it's a true emergency, what number they need to call and how they need to wake me up in the middle of the night because I won't get any email at night when I'm sleeping.

That's why I got the Apple Watch. When it first came out, I thought, "Why would I get this? What would I use it for?" And then when I opened up my concierge boutique-type practice, I realized, "Wow, I get hundreds of emails a day. I have to be able to know the ones that are important for me to look at and respond right away." So on my Apple Watch I get alerted for patient emails, phone calls through my office or phone calls from my immediate family. Everything else will just go straight to my cell phone and sit there.

There's a lot of talk that the Apple Watch doesn't have that "killer app" yet, but you're saying it's valuable for you in your practice simply by having email alerts. It doesn't sound like it has to be revolutionary to improve patient communication.

Right. The one thing that I did learn which I think is important to know is that it will only notify you when it's on your wrist. If you take it off and it's charging next to you on your nightstand, it will not alert you because it's activated when it's on your wrist. It took me a few nights to realize that.

What types of information do you find engaging to your followers? Are they asking for more wellness tips and medical advice?

Sometimes I write a blog and I'll send that out. I might be speaking locally and so I'll put that on my office Facebook or Twitter. But in general, a lot of it is what I am reading and information that I am finding out there, which could be written by another pediatrician or a top mommy blogger and I think, "Wow, this is a really great article." I want to share it with my followers, with my patients, with my readers and then I send it out there.

What is your social media strategy?

Once I went to a lecture on how to use Twitter and Facebook and, I guess, become "popular" and get followers in whatever your specialty is. They actually had guidelines that you should send out something every hour, like five a day of things that you've written, five a day things that other people have written.

    I am so busy in a given day seeing patients, dealing with my own children, working on my books, blogs and news segments that I don't really think about how many I've sent out or, "Did I not even send anything out today?" It's just more when I come across things that I find valuable or if I'm getting a lot of questions from parents on a specific topic that day, I will look for a resource and then put it out there so my families and others can get the information.

Is it important for your posts to be authentic so that it's obvious a human being is on the other end of the feed?

Yes, exactly. You can probably tell when I'm in between patients because I might push out three things at once and then you won't hear from me for four hours.

Why is it important to consider their families when you're talking with patients?

Well, I think the family is very important when it comes to kids. If you're talking about nutrition, sleep, screen time, it doesn't only affect the patient on your table, but it affects everybody else in the house. So if the parents have good habits and they're healthy, that's going to trickle down to the child's health. Also with illnesses, if I'm taking care of, let's say, a child with strep throat, for example, I'm not going to only focus on that child.

Then I always turn to the parents and I say, "Okay, this is what you want to do in the house to decrease the chance that anyone else will get it. These are the signs that you want to look for if you or dad start to have a sore throat or a fever or if the baby seems really fussy. Those are signs that any of you might have contracted strep, then you need to call me and come into the office so we can swab you." You always want to look beyond that patient on the table and see what else you can do to educate the family.

You know what's interesting is now that I'm in private solo practice, everyone says, "Don't patients bug you all the time?" You can't share a call with anybody. But honestly, I feel that I educate my families so well, I rarely get called after hours and I have not been woken up in the middle of the night, knock on wood, since I opened my own practice just a few months ago.

So at least in your experience with the new private practice, you are able to make it work for you in a similar way to email? And it isn't too time-consuming?

Exactly. By educating the patients and their families, I'm proactively addressing a lot of their questions they would be calling me for after hours, but I have a good idea of what some of those questions are going to be in advance. So I think those are definitely keys to engage with not just patients but everyone who's involved with them.

Because I'm only seeing a dozen patients a day instead of 40, any very sick child or anyone that I'm concerned about, I will call them in the evening or email them at night and say, "Okay, this is what you're going to do if X, Y and Z happens" and we come up with a plan ahead of time, that way I'm not going to sleep saying, "I hope that child doesn't spike a high fever at night. I hope they don't throw up again."

I've already given the parents clear instructions on what we're going to do if all these things happen that I know since I've been doing this for 15 years now what might potentially happen with this child and with this illness. Then I also let them know that they should call me and wake me up. Although usually I've helped them already and educated them so well that that's not going to happen. But just in case, I always give them that last line, "It's okay to call and wake me up if . . ."

Does it offends you when patients and families research their own conditions and bring those questions to you?

There is so much information available now for families that in some ways, they can be their own doctor or their own health advocate and they can Google the symptoms that their child has, and a good amount of the time actually figure out what is going on. In some cases they can get really great instructions on what to do and how to treat their child.

Where you do need to be a little careful is there's also a lot of not-great information out there on the Internet, as we know, especially when it comes to certain topics like vaccines. So I try to direct my families to my favorite sites. Once I had a mom say, "I always type in what I'm looking for and I'll type in your name and I'll get some article you were interviewed with or some news segment or something you wrote and then at least I know that it's accurate if your name is attached to it." I thought that was funny. But I have not covered every topic out there, obviously.

I like when parents call me and they have knowledge and they're educated. It makes the conversation more interesting when you can talk to them on a different level. That said, it's also important to remember that this is a parent who likely did not go to medical school. And even though they may think that they know everything, you still want to take a step back and sort of reeducate them and fill in the little gaps so that way you don't find out later on like, "I actually didn't understand that," or, "I didn't realize that," or, "I wasn't thinking about that," or, "I thought you said the fever was okay, that's why I didn't call you when it was lasting seven days."

So you always want to say even though with the flu, you may have a fever for five days, if it goes on day six or seven or it goes away and then it comes back, that's a reason you need to come into the office and I need to actually listen to your child and check them out.

There is another way that I like to use the Internet. For example, I was skiing with my family a few weekends ago. A family that comes to my office called me and said that their daughter had a rash. We talked about what it might be.

I said, "Do you have a computer in front of you? Why don't you look up pityriasis rosea. Does this kind of look like what your teenage daughter has? Because that's what I'm thinking based on what you described to me. It's not dangerous. I'm going to be back in the office in two days. I can take a look at it then. I don't think you need to rush to an urgent care. But if for some reason she starts not feeling well, having any swelling, any bruising, high fevers, then you do need to go to the urgent care and be seen, otherwise it can wait two days."

Sure enough, they looked it up and although the mom wasn't sure, the teenage daughter was like, "Definitely, Mom, that's what my rash looks like." So I think it can also be a tool for us to better help our families when we're not able to see them face to face.

8
POSITION DIGITAL MARKETING EXPERTS TO LEAD
A CONVERSATION WITH AARON WATKINS

In this chapter, you will learn why it's important to create health care content for patients and make it easy to find online. Aaron Watkins is senior director of Internet strategy & digital content marketing at Johns Hopkins Medicine. I invited him on the program after hearing him speak at HCIC (the Health Care Internet Conference). He has worked for years to blow the doors off of organizational silos in one of the world's most renowned academic medical institutions. A hospital or practice's digital marketing team has a vested interest in working with clinicians to create and optimize health literacy and patient education materials. These same guidelines apply whether working with an in-house digital marketing team or an outside resource.

What have you learned as you have attempted to socialize the web strategy within your organization?

What I really want to do is connect in all of our leaders' minds the understanding that the web is a huge part of patient experience. It is, in many cases, the only brand touch point they'll have with us because we have a goal to educate people around the world. It's just the key experience point of anyone who's engaging us. I really work to communicate that.

When I started in this role, I was really frustrated. I felt like I bring a lot of expertise. I've been doing this, building websites and doing it since the mid '90s. But what I found was a lot of people working independently and not really wanting to listen. I was really frustrated and talked to a successful executive in DC whom I met through a networking group. He said, "Don't be so hard on yourself. If you've said something 29 times, you're just getting warmed up."

That really resonated with me. I realized we really have to work as educators in our institutions and keep repeating the same things and keep looking for those people with whom it resonates and who can then start to collaborate. I found that once I started doing that, it was actually a lot easier. I used to go in and really show lots of data and just share all the great things we were doing. But really you have to be patient and look for the opportunities to establish that you're working for common goals.

As an example, findability of content is our biggest challenge as an organization. That reflects what a big enterprise we are. It goes to our core goal of my team. We definitely want a great search experience. We want HopkinsMedicine.org at the top of search engines. When people are on our site, we want them to get to the information that they need.

But when I first started, people didn't seem to realize that. They would tell me we're not doing well enough on search. It was an argument. I would sit back and instead of leading with data I started to learn to wait and hear what things people would bring up.

If they start talking about frustration that they're not at the top of search for a certain thing, that's when I jump in and talk about, "You're absolutely right. Findability of information is our key problem and here's what we're doing to address that kind of thing."

So I think the core message is focus on the simplest of problems and establish those common goals before you go in and do anything else in a conversation.

How does the digital marketing team get clinical buy-in for online content?

I used to assume that people really understood Johns Hopkins Medicine, that if you're a faculty member, whether you're research, clinical, or usually both, if you're an executive, you have a complete view. The reality is a lot of people are working in a silo. After a few years of being here, I found I'd actually presented to committees that some of our faculty had never even heard of.

It solidified when I was hearing our faculty express concerns that I can actually inform them not just about the web but about what is happening in other aspects of the organization. I try and play that support role whenever I can and try and build relationships within the organization whenever I can.

Another key thing I found, is a lot of health care organizations have a meeting-heavy culture. When you look at an organization like this, there are a lot of leaders. There are a lot of people making hard decisions every day and acting on that, perhaps with little information at that point in time. It's often in the context of a meeting where they're on stage. People are looking to them to be that leader and make that decision.

I try to do two things in that case. One, I try and socialize ideas before we get into those meetings. I try and make the connection with the person who I anticipate will be the decision-maker in that meeting, whether that is a faculty member, an administrator, an executive, whoever it may be. I try to talk to them first and share what information we're going to bring.

I really try and support their goals, listen to the things that are on their minds, and adjust. I try to avoid a situation where we're forcing anyone to make a decision that they might be uncomfortable with because when that happens most people fall back on a prior decision. They want to look consistent.

So if in the past they haven't collaborated with our web team in any way, that's probably where they're going to land again. Again, you've got to build those relationships coming into the room and you've got to try to avoid putting anyone in a situation where they have to make a quick decision without the information and in a way that they feel like their reputation in some way is on the line in front of their peers.

Why is it important to do user testing and challenge assumptions?

We've done numerous tests on our content over the years and evolved how we approach it. A few years ago we did a study that was really pivotal to how we approach health content. We had a doctor who wanted to share a ton of information. He also had just two pieces of information that he wanted people to remember, one of which he considered critical. "If they know this then they'll probably decide to take action and probably with me," he reasoned.

We presented it how he had written it on the website. We went out to do a user test. We had an incredibly low retention of that piece of information that he wanted to share. We did another round of testing where we just moved it up. We put it in a box. Basically, we created this box that we call the "what you need to know" box. It had a few bullets in it.

What we found at the end when we tested for retention was that we increased that retention by more than 58%. Once we found that, we started approaching almost all of our health pages that way. You'll almost always see some form of a box with just two, three or four points that you need to know. It's great. It's almost a "get out of jail free" card in some ways for us because, one, it gives us credibility with the faculty to communicate it. But, two, it also gives us some ability to deal with longer forms of their content and share that below the page with a little more ability to edit it and guide them as well.

The biggest foundation of all of our research is an on-site survey on HopkinsMedicine.org. It gives us responses from all of our audiences, which is fantastic. When I'm meeting with someone who's concerned about education, I can say, "Well, here is what students are saying about our website. Here's what applicants to the med school are saying about the website." Similarly, I can talk about patients and caregivers. I've got great data sets for all of our key audiences.

Lastly, we do some market research as well. We've tried to understand how do people decide. Why did they decide to come to a certain doctor? Why did they decide to come to a certain hospital? How much do rankings play into it?

How much is it about the doctor and the information they

see? How much is it about what their peers are saying or what they're seeing in online reviews? We do a good deal of research on those topics and share that internally.

9
BUILD AN ONLINE COMMUNITY
A CONVERSATION WITH JOHN LYNN

In this chapter, you will learn about using blogging as a way to share your message, how changing reimbursement models are affecting care and how to create online communities. John Lynn is the founder and editor of HealthcareScene.com, the nationally renowned blog network with more than 10,000 articles that have been viewed over 17 million times. He's also the co-founder of the Health IT Marketing and PR Conference, or HITMC. I invited John on the program because he is a community builder, and because he packs a lot of wisdom in a short amount of time. The tips he has learned in building a health IT community apply to patient communities as well. He also builds a strong case for the value of clinicians getting more involved and familiar with health IT.

What can other health care audiences learn from the evolution of the health IT marketing community?

It's pretty interesting because if you look even, say, three years ago, there really wasn't a community. There were plenty of health care IT marketers. In fact, I describe it as the golden age of health IT marketing. We had $36 billion of stimulus money thanks to the RS stimulus package, or as we know it in health care, the High Tech Act which stimulated EHRs and everything associated with them. So it was a really exciting time for health IT marketing.

Everyone was kind of busy working in their siloes. They'd be going to conferences and certainly they were all at the same conferences, but when a marketer goes to a conference, they're going there managing all their people, managing the sales people, managing what coverage they're getting from media organizations and they're never talking to the people in the booths next to them. Matter of fact, maybe their salespeople or some of their leaders get to talk to them more than the marketing people because they're dealing with all sorts of event-related logistics, which make their job hard. So they really didn't connect with each other.

If you look even three years ago, there wasn't a community. These health IT marketers were doing their job and they were doing the best they could and occasionally they might meet one or two of their colleagues at these events or they'd connect with them in some other way. But they didn't really have a way to connect with each other.

Over the past couple years we've really seen a coming together, and I've actually seen this in many industries. It makes sense this happened in the marketing community as well, through social media, Twitter in particular, but also LinkedIn to some extent and other platforms like it that have helped the community to really come together. Obviously in my experience with HITMC, the Health IT Marketing Conference, that was another level of bringing the community together. It's been interesting to see the evolution.

Over these three years we've seen a community come together where one didn't exist before. In fact, that's the most exciting thing. If you look at other health care communities, there certainly have been other health care PR conferences and health care marketing conferences. We're similar in a lot of ways because we have HIPAA regulations. There are things we can't say. There are things we can say. We have to be careful about taking pictures at our venues.

I remember one of the early topics when the community was coming together was, "Where can I take some pictures of the hospital environment without getting patients there?" People gave you four or five simulation areas and different places they could go that weren't a HIPAA violation. Some of those kinds of things you have to deal with, even pharma and medical device regulations about what you promise and how you promise it. You have to deal with all of those things, so in some ways those are very similar.

For the most part it's quite a bit different though because in health care IT in particular, you're focused on very hard-to-reach people. You're talking about doctors, practice managers, hospital executives, hospital CIOs or hospital IT managers or maybe an HIM manager. So it's a very different approach than, say, a hospital that wants to market their hospital to patients, which is more of a consumer-focused play as opposed to more of the B2B focus, which most health IT companies have.

So I think those are some of the things we've seen and some of the differences we've seen.

What is the future of health care blogging?

It's quite interesting. We've seen a massive evolution over 10 years, as you can imagine. Ten years ago Twitter didn't even exist. Facebook was a college network and LinkedIn was your résumé. It didn't have groups or anything else. So we've seen this massive change in how people consume content and how they connect with other people.

Ten years ago, blogging was the way to connect with other people in the industry. So you would connect on the blog and the blog would essentially be a community of users, including the comments, including new people who would start a blog because they're like, "Oh, I want to connect with other people." Now we don't see that as much, unfortunately, because people are doing it on Twitter, LinkedIn, Facebook or other social media.

In some ways that's good because obviously it's easy for anyone to get involved with Twitter and start connecting. I'm a massive Twitter user with far too many accounts, so I understand it fully.

The thing that makes me sad about it, though, is that even though it's easier to get a message out on a lot of these, it doesn't have nearly the lasting impact. The time it takes you to write 140-character thing is very little, so you don't put as much effort into what you actually put out and it also is very short-lived. Once you've tweeted it out, it's gone. Whereas if you'd written a blog post about that same topic, those blog posts last much longer and they create a deeper connection between you the person you're connecting with.

I guess that's my sadness about some blogs. I used to call them my blog spar, where we would take a topic and we would essentially spar. I would write a blog post on one angle and then someone else would write a blog post arguing the other angle. Then I would reply again and kind of this spar match where we educated each other and we felt deeply about certain topics. Now that doesn't really happen too much. Occasionally but not very much because it's all happening on Twitter, it's happening on LinkedIn, other places.

But the thing that I think won't change is that people's desire to learn and share what they know will never disappear. That's just going to be a feature that we've always had. Ever since the days when you chiseled it into a rock, you wanted to share what you had and found. You'd put it on scrolls and have someone run a marathon over to the next city to share.

We have this insatiable need to share and also to learn, we want opportunities to learn. So I don't think that will ever go away. Just the modalities that we use to share that knowledge are going to change, and the technology we use to connect and share is going to change as well. But we'll always have a need for high-quality thought leadership and ways to improve what you do at work to improve what your organization can do to be more successful. So I think that will just always be there and there will always be a place for it.

The key is what's the right information to share and how are you going to get readers to read it? It's really a simple model when you look at the blogging model. You have to create amazing content. You have to market it so you get readers. Then you monetize it.

It's always been the media model. If you have people's attention, you can use some of that attention and provide opportunities for them to purchase something.

One thing I think has changed dramatically in blogging is how you approach what you sell. We're doing a lot of sponsored content, for example; with companies it's been a powerful thing and many people are afraid of sponsored content. But you have to realize that, like I said, this is a complex sell in health care IT and so the best way to sell to someone is to show that you know what you're talking about. If you know what you're talking about and you show that you're experienced in that, then they'll come to you and say, "Okay, tell me more." Then you'll have an opportunity to sell them.

So you'll build that relationship with them and you'll position yourself as a thought leader in the space. Then you'll have the opportunity to sell them, as opposed to trying to put up a banner which tries to get them somehow to recognize your brand or to purchase it.

Now, banner ads might be a great way to reinforce what you're doing in thought leadership and in content marketing so that then they're like, "Oh, I remember those five other things that they sent me that showed they know what they're talking about. Now I need your solutions so now I'll click the banner ad." We've seen that evolution where they're really providing great content and to me, blogging is the simplest form to publish online, so that's why blogging has always been so powerful.

What do you see in the next 2-3 years in health IT?

It's actually important for marketing too because marketers need to spend more time understanding what industry trends are so they know what the reporters want to write about, so they know what the customers cared about. So I think that's a great question even for marketers.

Speaking more generally, the biggest trend I see happening across all of health care in a variety of ways, is really the changing reimbursement models. I think doctors are scared about what's happening. Sure we had this fix that came, but all that did was, okay, fine, we're not going to give you your 22% decrease in Medicare reimbursement which had been hanging over their head forever and everyone knew that was never going to happen.

But instead what they gave as a concession is that now you've got to change to value-based reimbursement. Unfortunately, most of health care has no idea what that is. In fact, I'm not sure anyone in health care knows what that is. We're still trying to figure it out.

These changing reimbursement models are going to change so much of how organizations act and that's true of hospitals, that's true of the small doctors' offices. Some people are making the case that the small doctors' offices are going to die because of it. They won't be able to keep up, that they'll have to join in some sort of consortium or get bought up by the hospital system in order to do a value-based reimbursement model.

Those things are going to drastically change what people purchase, how they purchase, when they purchase, and it influences almost everything in health care IT because health care IT is going to be required to facilitate these reimbursement models. Meaningful Use has kind of run its course. We know where that spending is essentially going, so now they're looking at what's next and I think it's these changing reimbursement models that are going to really impact it a lot.

Related to that is the ACA stuff with health insurance exchanges, which is a totally different legislation, even though many in the industry like to write about them being the same thing—Meaningful Use versus ACA, versus this change in reimbursement models like ACOs. There's a new acronym every week it seems.

But the other one with ACA, with Obamacare if you prefer, is that we're seeing a lot more patients with high deductible plans. As a matter of fact, I've seen study after study after study showing this. We're seeing this in practices where a lot of these patients that are coming in with health insurance exchange plans that they've gotten through Obamacare or through some other are coming in as high deductible plans and they don't even realize it.

So what does that mean if they have a high deductible plan? That means the patient's going to pay a lot more, the insurance is going to pay a lot less and these patients aren't ready to pay for it. So you can imagine how that changing environment is going to impact care. I heard it from Intermountain, a large, massive hospital system across all of Utah. What do they own? Some massive percentage of health care in Utah. They're saying the same thing.

They're seeing massive shifts to patient pay versus insurance pay, and their collections rate with patients is so much lower than insurances, so that's hitting their bottom line. Then along with that change is patients now care a lot more about what they're buying. Since I'm going to have to pay more, I may or may not take that service or I may be more interested in shopping around for my doctor.

It changes how you handle health care when you start paying for it. These changes and models are really going to impact people's purchasing decisions. On the negative side, doctors are scared. On the positive side from a marketing standpoint is if you have a solution that can solve that problem, it's a tremendous opportunity because technology is going to be the way that many of these problems are solved and many of these problems are attacked, with technology. Probably with a mix of humans as well, but it's a tremendous opportunity if you can solve that.

So I would look at this, ACOs, value-based reimbursement, high deductible insurance plans with patient self-pay and things like that, and as many things are happening that health care IT will need to solve.

10
HEALTH CARE IS ALWAYS PERSONAL
A CONVERSATION WITH LINDA STOTSKY

In this chapter, you will learn how to consider and stand up for patient advocates. Linda Stotsky is a health IT usability analyst and was named in the top 5 of the 2016 #HIT100. I invited Linda on the program because of her personal experiences as a patient advocate since before it was a movement. Between her mother, her daughter and her son, she has been a patient advocate over several different types of care, aging care, disorders, as well as disease. You will find her personal perspective refreshing and insightful.

What is patient advocacy?

Patient advocacy involves the voice of the patient within navigating the health care ecosystem and understanding the challenges, treatment planning, diagnosis and care management. There's a need for patient advocates, in continuing care settings in the hospital as inpatients as well as outpatient.

There's a large continuum of patient advocacy. I think it begins with understanding medical jargon and understanding what's at stake in terms of decision making. It also means helping patients when they're more vulnerable and they don't have the ability to speak up regarding choices in care; also medical and/or coordination of care.

Where do you see the greatest opportunities in patient advocacy?

We have an enormous opportunity in the industry to make sure that all patients can access their medical records, they understand the information that's presented in medical jargon and they are informed about disease management choices.

IT system vendors have an opportunity to include the patient voice in design discussions, development and educational materials. There are many opportunities for patient participation in national studies regarding health issues. I see a lot of advisory boards enlarging to include patients. I believe that patient advocacy will grow tremendously in the next five years or so.

We need advocates who can navigate the health care ecosystem and have an understanding of regulatory, compliant and clinical aspects so that they can understand the critical next steps in the process and become a valuable asset to caregivers.

What do clinicians need to know to help patient advocacy?

From a clinical standpoint we have to realize that we can't just incorporate a patient portal and expect all patients to understand results, lab tests, medical choices and information. We need to customize the information so that it fits the needs of the patient.

It must fit their needs on a literacy level and be presented in living room language. In other words when we exchange information and provide data to patients, such as lab results, we need a standard way to improve our translation of the results so that patients understand what the values mean.

A good rule of thumb test is naming tests in a way that corresponds with what system they include. In other words HDL and LDL become high and low cholesterol. There's a really simple way to communicate information to patients in a way they understand. Right now I think we're connecting results with patient portals, but we're missing that critical step of translating the information in a way that makes sense to the patient, so they take those values forward to make changes in their lives.

What are the greatest challenges in patient advocacy?

I may be going against what I just said, but I think the greatest challenge is in turning requests into actionable change within the health care enterprise. Again, while we advocate for patient portals and patient access to medical information, we have to make sure that the information we're translating and the information we're providing can be used in an actionable way.

The ability to be heard is a huge problem right now in health care for patient advocates. We're a long way from a two-way relationship between patients and providers. We are not sensitive to patient values and input. We need actionable strategy to embrace the patient and their family as partners both in the diagnosis and treatment planning, and also in future care management. I think there's a need for more advocates and more patient navigators in complementary settings such as long term care, rehabilitation, pediatrics and hospice.

Sometimes we're brought into the mix when the situation is already adversarial. We're promoting or advocating for the patient just during that adversarial confrontation. It becomes somewhat of a confrontation. What we need is a greater effort by the medical community as a whole to include those patient voices and patient advocates as part of the conversation before it becomes adversarial.

While a lot of hospitals are hiring patient advocates right now, I'm not so sure that this is the way to go about it because once you have a financial stake in the employee, there's somewhat of a conflict right there in their advocacy. Can they be candid? Can they be forthright? Can they speak without retribution? It's a tricky mix. I think we need to continue to challenge prevention, how to prevent actions before they occur, and how to fully rectify a situation without becoming adversarial so that the patient experience is improved overall.

Is there resistance to patient advocacy, and if so, what do we do to help overcome that?

We need to listen. The two-way conversations are somewhat muted on the listening side. I was recently with my daughter. She underwent surgery. While we were in the recovery room, it was unbelievable to me how frustrating it was as her biggest supporter to just get people to listen to me. If she had been by herself during this experience, I'm sure that her health and the time that she spent in the hospital would have been compromised.

We need a larger conversation between primary care and secondary care. We need care coordination to be a broader part of our strategy in improving the quality of care delivery. We have to improve these communication channels, so that when we have conflict and situations that need tighter coordination and more communication; we are listened to.

I find it very frustrating because after the experience with my daughter I reached out to some C-Suite friends at the hospital, actual friends of mine. I basically explained the situation that happened, the gaps and the critical components that were missing. I didn't even get an answer. Did anyone care? (These are really close friends.)

I shudder to think about the patient or the patient advocate that doesn't have these inroads and who doesn't have the ability to write an email or doesn't know the email address. We need health care organizations to listen to these real-life situations and include patients in two-way conversation.

You've said that not much has changed in terms of care coordination, with all of the technology and systems we use today. What changes would you like to see in the next five years?

One thing I would like to see is a larger communication channel. We don't communicate well past the physical walls of a facility. When we're exchanging information, many times critical information is incomplete and incomplete information results in medical error and hospital re-admission.

I believe we need to tighten up both at the micro level and the macro level. We need to look at our protocols. Many times patients experience infection due to incomplete protocols at the facility level. There should be a macro-level integration with the facility and a micro-level improvement in the clinical guidelines and protocols within our EHR systems.

These protocols don't need to interrupt or provide additional noise or alerts, but rather intuitively recognize gaps and improve the transition to reminders and checklists. I think the difference in care protocols from one facility to another causes critical gaps. These gaps can be accompanied by physical changes in the patient such as delirium, psychosomatic changes, pain and decompensation before the readmission cycle.

It has been 15 years since I experienced this with my mother. Yet when I accompanied my neighbor's father through his transfer from an inpatient facility to a long-term care facility, I saw the exact same behavior repeated, resulting in the same infection and ending with his readmission to the hospital.

I saw a quote from George Bernard Shaw that reads, "The single biggest problem with communication is the illusion that it's taking place." We've come a long way with technology, but sometimes we find it difficult to initiate a conversation. This can be as simple as picking up the phone in certain situations. Within the next five years I want to see a better way to open up communication channels—especially during transitions of care.

-II-
USING DIGITAL HEALTH TOOLS

11
THE EARLY ADOPTER ADVANTAGE
A CONVERSATION WITH DR. WEN DOMBROWSKI
AND FARD JOHNMAR

In this chapter, you will learn the results of the 2016 State of Digital Health Innovation survey and what they mean for clinicians. Dr. Wen Dombrowski is a physician informaticist and digital innovation strategist with clinical expertise in the care of medically complex and socially complex patients. Fard Johnmar is the president and CEO of Enspektos, who facilitated the study. The study revealed some enlightening statistics: only 5% of health systems are operating at a peak level of digital health innovation, and even when they are working on value-based initiatives as an organization, the C-suite is often still focused on legacy sources of revenue. Fard and Dr. Donbrowski dig into the implications of today's transformation in care and how clinicinas can take advantage.

What are the top takeaways from the study, and what was the most surprising?

(Fard) The top takeaway from the State of Digital Health Innovation Study is that only 5% of health organizations globally are operating at peak digital health innovation efficiency. So basically it means that a lot of organizations are trying to sustain their innovations, make sure they're funded appropriately and measure them appropriately.

In this particular study, we looked at some very important forces that are impacting digital health innovation. Through that process, the respondents to the study and the respondents to this data were people working within health organizations, government agencies, pharmaceutical companies, payers, hospitals, as well as their partners, people who were coming into these organizations and helping the people from the health organizations execute.

By bringing together insights from both those points of view, we're basically finding that not just in the U.S., but also around the world, the results were consistent around the world that many organizations are having a difficult time scaling and diffusing their innovations internally and externally.

So why is this idea of scaling and diffusing innovation really important and why is it that I decided to focus on that 5% statistic? We have a challenge currently in health care in the U.S. and globally. The challenge is how do we take and use these digital innovations that people are talking about a great deal and are very excited about and have the potential to really transform health and use them in ways that are going to be appropriate for physicians for patients and really solve some of the deepest and most pressing issues that we face in health care today?

If we're going to be able to do that successfully using these technologies, we really do need to do a better job of implementing around digital health.

(Wen) In my experience, I've spoken to a number of innovation leaders in health systems across the country; I've also worked with a number of different health systems. One of the barriers to executing digital health successfully is the lack of alignment at the C-suite level; that includes commitment to financial investment, commitment to changing the operational workflow processes and then also changing the organizational culture. That is fundamentally needed in order to change the way things have always been done.

In the forward to the study, you wrote, "Some changes may temporarily cannibalize legacy sources of revenue, but there are significant first mover advantages." What are the early adopter advantages to digital health?

First I'd like to start with some background related to the legacy sources of revenue that are preventing the alignment towards the new digital health innovations. For many decades, most hospitals and other health care provider organizations have focused their business models on maximizing the number of patients that physically go to their hospitals, ER's or doctor's offices.

When I speak with my colleagues in other health systems, most of the health systems, even the ones that have announced that they're working on innovation or value-based care initiatives, often times their C-suite is very focused on the fee for service mentality of maximizing the physical visits and therefore, they're not necessarily willing to invest financially and do the operational changes and culture changes needed.

So one of the things that I've noticed is that a lot of times it's easy for leaders of any organization to get caught in the trap of thinking that, "We've been successful for the past ten years, so of course we will be successful the next ten years." This resting on the laurels of past success is very dangerous, but very common and prevalent in health care organizations.

What we're seeing in recent years is that, especially in small and medium-sized organizations, they're starting to go through financial distress or be acquired because of their reliance on past successes. I know there are large organizations that will say they're too big to fail. But even large organizations are susceptible to the market forces and consumer forces that are changing the nature of the game.

I'm seeing this with a lot of health care organizations, whether it's providers or some payers or pharmaceutical and device companies, depending on the companies. It's not necessarily all organizations, but a large number of them are failing to recognize the rapidly evolving market forces, consumer demands and technology enablers.

The game is changing and the rules of the game are different. Think about an all-star football player that became famous for his ability to play football but he may not know how to play soccer or how to successfully compete in a soccer match.

Bringing this analogy back to health care, when we see health care executives resting on their laurels of past success, they're focusing on maximizing hospitalizations, surgeries and office visits. That is what the old and current reimbursement system rewards but not necessarily what's going to be successful in the coming year and upcoming years.

So going back to your original question about first mover advantage, what I'm seeing is that patients increasingly want more convenience and personalized services. Also, outside of the consumer space, there are increasingly more technologies that enable any competitor of health care to really deliver what their consumers want in a new way.

For example, if someone isn't feeling well in the middle of the night or if they're at work and they're not feeling well, they don't necessarily have the time or the energy to drive across town to see a doctor. So something like a telemedicine urgent care service would be helpful not only to these patients, but it can also drive new sources of revenue and customer acquisition to the health care providers.

In this scenario, when the person is not feeling well, often times they might search on Google to ask what should they do or where should they go to get help. I believe the telemedicine services that are proactively available in the market will appear in the search results in the ads. Whichever one that the consumer clicks first, not only does that telemedicine company benefit from that one customer interaction, but that telemedicine company has the potential to determine all the subsequent referrals and utilization.

For example, if a patient sees a telemedicine provider online, that provider determines the patient needs further follow up, that provider has the ability to refer the patient to a specific provider network of ambulances, ER, surgeons, dermatologists, laboratories and other services. So they're really affecting not just that one time point of care interaction, but the customer lifetime value and their entire subsequent network utilization.

I think that organizations that can think about this immediate and future competitive advantage are already investing in the technical, human and marketing capabilities to launch these types of services locally. What's interesting is that unlike old forms of health care where launching health care services was very much only a local play, now companies that can build a technology-enabled electronic or digital service not only are able to reach their local markets, but then they have the ability to scale to wider geographies and become competitive entrants into new markets.

How can clinicians move forward and embrace digital health?

(Fard) I think the type of comments that Wen has been making are really critical in terms of moving away from the "shock and awe" of digital health to the nuts and bolts of digital health. Overall, digital health is moving into what I call the Age of Implementation.

One of the things that we saw over the last year is that the types of topics that the people were referring to regarding implementation including conducting research and testing digital health tools are becoming more part of the conversation as we move on. That was just looking at about 630,000 social media data points.

So that speaks to the fact that a lot of people are thinking about the issues that Wen has been discussing. How do we change from an older revenue model that focused on volume to a newer revenue model that's focused on value? How do we take advantage of the ways that consumers in particular are utilizing these technologies in order to access things like entertainment and food and really having an expectation that health care is going to operate in the same way.

But at the same time that they're thinking through these challenges, the big question is how can we as an organization really try to figure out how to overcome or deal with the barriers? These transformations are difficult. In some cases, payer organizations can bring on certain types of initiatives that may have an impact on their regulatory posture, or their exposure to certain compliance and regulations can really have a big impact on the speed to innovation.

So people often ask why it takes a major payer or a hospital sometimes a year and a half to go from learning about an innovation to actually executing. It's because of the fact that people within the organization really need to be thinking through these policy and regulatory-related issues or dealing with what I call the human issues in terms of leadership support or also dealing with the economic issues, right? How do you engage in activities that are going to save money for the institution or actually make money?

Finally, how do you deal with those technological issues in terms of what it actually takes to deploy? So when you think about the impact of what I call those forces shaping digital health innovation, and again, that information is in the research report, it becomes very clear that even though people are moving toward focusing on this implementation issue, that it's not the sexiest conversation to have.

But it's the one that we need to be having in order to move from this posture of hoping that somehow digital will be transformative to actually doing the things that we need to do to make sure that is.

Finally, I'll talk about what this means for clinicians. One of the things that I hear in speaking with clinicians is they're often times blindsided in some respects by all of these new technologies, all of these new workflows that are being imposed on how they work as a physician. I think physicians really should have a voice in how these technologies are being deployed and the ways they're going to be touching patients and others.

12
REDUCE THE BARRIERS TO ENTRY
A CONVERSATION WITH DR. RICHARD MILANI

In this chapter, you will learn how a health system took seriously its responsibility to improve the health of its population by bringing apps to its patients. Dr. Richard Milani is chief clinical transformation officer for Ochsner Health. I invited him on the program because I want more clinicians to know about the O Bar, the revolutionary in-person patient engagement experience inside Ochsner's hospitals. Their clinical team approached challenges of bringing mobile health to patients who are elderly or less tech-savvy, even when there are 110,000 health and wellness apps out there. They also started with the attitude that they ultimately need to enhance the health of the population we serve. Dr. Milani has embraced his role as a change agent, and the result is progress toward achieving the elusive triple aim.

Tell us about your role as chief clinical transformation officer. Has that existed for a while in your organization?

I am the first one to hold that title in our organization and it's a relatively new role, even on a national scale, but there are others that I have met that are in the same type of role. So I think it speaks to the fact that health care is undergoing great transformation and we really need somebody who wakes up and thinks about nothing more than how we can improve how we care for patients and create not only efficiencies on the caregiver side, but better access and better outcomes on the patient side as well.

Our role is to try and invent and innovate new ways of both delivering care and improving care across the patients that we serve. We have innovation programs in terms of care delivery models both on the inpatient and the outpatient side, and many of them are using technology to be able to not only improve safety and improve care and better outcomes, but also improve caregiver efficiency, so when possible to try and utilize technology to improve care overall.

The O Bar is basically a genius bar in a physical location where patients are able to work with staff to have apps put on their mobile devices. What problems does it solve?

First, let's describe the issues and then how O Bar could be a solution. One issue is that there currently are about 110,000 health and wellness apps out there in the universe and there have been a couple of studies that found that there are some that are really very, very helpful and some may be moderately helpful, and some that are probably not too valuable at all. So that's one issue.

So how does the average consumer that doesn't have a health

background separate the wheat from the chaff so to speak, to discern which ones would be the better suited for them?

Then the second issue that really does exist is one of technology and, to some extent, even technophobia. It certainly may be perceived as a complex nature of technology, and it can be a barrier to many people that would benefit from technology.

A great example, and I'm not trying to be stereotypical or disparaging, but often older individuals sometimes will develop technophobia or a fear of certain new technologies because they're not used to it, so much so that even the AARP, the American Association of Retired Persons, has actually put around the country what they call "tech workshops," which are workshops where older individuals as part of AARP could understand how to do what you and I might consider relatively routine things, whether it be using a tablet or email or any of the number of apps and technologies that exist today for the average person.

So that's a way of sort of reducing the barrier to entry. It's reducing that hurdle. We felt that obviously technology can help a lot of people, especially those with chronic disease, for them to be able to get more involved in their own care, to not be so reliant always on the health system but to be able to take control or at least partial control over their own health.

So the idea was to be able to solve both those problems and that's where the O Bar was conceived. The O Bar is literally something kind of like the genius bar. It's a bar in a retail area. Not a bar where you drink obviously, but where we have half a dozen or so iPads that are mounted. We've loaded onto them several hundred apps that are broken down by category that subject matter experts have evaluated and felt that these are among the good ones.

So if you are a diabetic or you wanted to lose weight or you wanted to improve your nutrition or whatever it might be or issues around women's health or pregnancy or any of those kind of things, you'd have a curated set of apps that we know that probably has a good chance of being reasonably effective and that other patients have felt to be useful as well.

Secondly, there's a "genius" as you pointed out, an expert behind the bar, that can help and assist not only in guiding you, but should you have an issue with technology, they could take all the pain points away. They can load the app on your on your smartphone or tablet. They can help you in terms of the set up.

Now again, the kind of outcomes I can discuss with anybody listening is that they're anecdotes because, again, this is information that's held through HIPAA that we can't really go and access an individual's information. We've had many, many patients come to us and tell us how much an app or this kind of information has really changed their lives and how it's helped them accomplish things that they otherwise wouldn't have been able to accomplish.

How did you gain buy-in for the O Bar?

It first took a concept and some national survey data that suggested patients are interested in getting more involved in their own care. This was never meant to be, nor is it, a profitable venture. If anything, it's a money-losing venture if you look at it just in terms of dollars and cents. But we're not for profit, not that we're here to just throw money away, but the idea being is that we need to be enhancing the health of the population we serve.

We think that this is providing the capability for our patients to enhance their health and learn more about their own disease processes. So it is an investment that we make in our patients and that's the way we look at it. I'm very fortunate to have a very forward-thinking CEO and board of directors that embrace this and really felt it was a great experiment to try, and if it didn't work then no problem, but if it did, then all the better. Thus far it's been very successful for us. In fact, we're actually expanding the number of locations where we have O Bars.

So providers don't have to create a whole custom suite of apps that will take a considerable amount of time, resources and budget? They can work with the thousands of apps and connected devices that are already out there?

Absolutely. Think of it as opening up a library. You don't have to write all the books that are in the library. What you want to do is create a vehicle by which people can access the information held within the library, and that's really all this is. It's a resource guided by a librarian for lack of a better analogy, where we don't have to write the books. We don't have to write the apps or develop the technology. What we need to do is curate it and provide it in a way that makes it very easy to digest for our patients and we think can be helpful to them.

What do you say to clinicians who are still skeptical about using digital health apps or empowering patients?

I think we have to determine what the reasons are why they're skeptical. So is it because the information is not secure, or is the information not valid, or what I hear the most is that the information is too much. So that we have all this flood of data coming in, we don't know how we're going to possibly manage it. So the concern that I've heard the most often voiced is that the physician is burdened too much as it is, and now if you flood the physician, and particularly the primary care physician with this enormity of data, then how are we going to possibly manage that? I think that's an appropriate concern.

So this is how I think we need to reorganize ourselves from a care team perspective. We've created an IPU model, an integrated practice unit of non-physician care teams that help analyze the data and make interventions. So it's not a burden; it's actually a relief for the primary care physician (or whatever physician may be involved in the care of that patient). The data comes in and goes through an analytics engine. It goes through all those machinations that I referred to earlier, and then the analytics engine tells the care team, "These are people you need to be concerned about and these are the ones you want to focus in on today."

That care team, whether they be a clinical pharmacist or a health coach or a nurse, can then contact that patient and then make whatever appropriate interventions are necessary, including medication change or lifestyle recommendations or even an appointment for the clinic. So we've been able to manage the data very securely and security has not been an issue. We're using only HIPAA-compliant interfaces.

Certainly the information is available to anybody on the care team, including the physician any time they want to utilize it. So I think it's okay to be skeptical. We just have to address what the issues are specifically and show them how it can be utilized to make care more effective and more efficient.

13
TAME THE DATA BEAST
A CONVERSATION WITH DR. RASU SHRESTHA

In this chapter, you will learn what it means to be data rich but information poor and the fundamentals of what it means to leverage data to rethink health care. Dr. Rasu Shrestha is the chief innovation officer at UPMC and is a passionate hybrid of clinician and health IT innovator. I invited him on the program because his name kept coming up when I first became engaged in the health IT community. He participates often in Twitter chats, blogs and conferences. Dr. Shrestha's insightful look at the future of care sheds a great deal of light on how clinical teams need to advance past the culture of analog. In short, don't get so caught up in the regulations and traditions of today (the present) that you lose sight of why you went into medicine (the past) and the data revolution that is coming (the future).

What is your concept that we are data rich and information poor?

It's really interesting where we are as an industry. The last decade has been transformative for us in health care as we've moved from analog to digital. It's really important for us to connect big data to big insights. It's not just about having data, because often times we're drowning in data that we're generating across the board.

I wanted to give a wakeup call for us in health care to comprehend the power of data and to actively seek insights that can be garnered from all of the right purchases to primarily the big data technologies and things that we have at hand. In health care today, we're data rich and information poor. I say that as a clinician, I play more of a role of a detective than I do as a clinician because I'm always trying to piece information together.

So we're drowning in data, right? What's really interesting is 90% of all of the data in the world, even outside of health care, has really been generated over the last two years. We're seeing a tremendous influx of data. So how do we really leverage that data? How do we manage to go from data to insights and make sure we're able to put that data to work for us? Data is a big asset. So I've tried to really demystify what big data means and really try to look into the future of how we might be able to transform health care leveraging big data technologies.

How do we focus on insights, not data?

It's really important not to be blinded by buzzwords. You hear a lot of buzzwords out there. Big data, unfortunately, has become a buzzword and so have a lot of other things out there, like "pop health," for example. So when we think about big data, this need for us to tame the data beast is real.

I draw analogies to us being gardeners of big data. I think, much like how a gardener sows his seeds and cares and nurtures his garden, it's important for us to manage that data, especially when it's data at scale, with some level of discipline and a good deal of passion, right? It's important for us to have disciplined methodologies around data integration, data governance, data quality and security and information lifecycle management. We have a lot of data stewards at UPMC as we're trying to do the weeding and the pruning of the data.

As we look at these data farms, to take that analogy even out further, and we look at how the crops of data may yield insightful ingredients that we then cook up in the care processes that we're putting in place, it's important to make sure that we nurture the data in the right way. So it's not just a matter of let's go live with as many systems as possible and end up with all these silos of information systems that literally aren't talking to each other. It's really about this discipline of managing data intelligently and then get to that goal of having meaningful insights at the point of decision making.

How do we liberate data and make it useful?

I think it's really important for us to really take a step back, perhaps, and comprehend where we are as an industry. As we're looking forward in the space of health IT, it's important for us to understand the things we're able to dream up today could not really have been dreamt up even ten years ago. Today we've moved from analog to digital in large parts. There are still areas of focus that need to really embrace the digital form factor.

But we've got all these zeroes and ones in our servers, in the cloud, in our data centers, so it's really important to understand that data is an asset. But it's also important to understand that for us to fully generate value out of the asset, we need to liberate the data. Data liquidity is a phrase I use quite a bit to really draw upon the notion that data needs to be freed.

We celebrate when we go live with an electronic medical record or a specific system that we're deploying. There's good reason to celebrate, but I think that's the beginning of the journey; turning that system on and going live with it starts the data collection process. What's really important is to make sure that we're able to move up in that pyramid.

So at the bottom of the pyramid, which is really where we are in health care today, we've got all these siloes of information systems that aren't truly talking to each other in many ways. We're still trying to push the boundaries of interoperability.

How do we move from syntactic interoperability, which is pulling all of these systems together and connecting the pipes, to semantic data interoperability, where we look at semantic data harmonization and ontologies and the language behind these standards, whether it's SNOMED or LOINC or all of these systems that we have at the back end and translate and get to the meaning behind the data?

So semantic data harmonization becomes super important. But beyond that, it's also leveraging technologies like natural language processing. In health care, 80% of the data is unstructured data. So how do we go into the nitty-gritty details of radiology reports and discharge summaries and pathology reports and post-op notes? Beyond that even leveraging technologies like machine learning, where we have pattern recognition capabilities and deep learning capabilities to really decipher the signal from the noise and look at trends.

So that's how we really get to adding intelligence and insights to the data. Liberating the data has to become a strategic imperative for health care organizations across the board.

Why is it important to tell the story of innovation in health care?

We live in interesting times. I believe we're really in a smack of the dawn of this new era in health care, where the power of digital is just being comprehended. We're just at the dawn of that era. You remember when we had dial-up modems and the irritating yet satisfying sound of that dialup modem trying to latch onto the Internet and squeeze them away. Then you make that connection and then you're online.

You open up a web browser and type in hotmail.com. After a couple minutes, that first page opens up and you're celebrating. That's where we are in health care today when it comes to leveraging digital and leveraging the power of these algorithms and computerization today. We're just at that dawn.

And what's most interesting is that unlike with the dial-up modem, we won't have to wait decades for WiFi-enabled vehicles and fiber optic Internet to our homes. The future in health care is coming at a much quicker pace than it's ever come before. That makes it really interesting.

But it also brings these challenges of how do we make sure that this progress that we've made in the last decade-plus and moving from analog to digital and moving from film to filmless and paper to paperless, how do we make sure we don't repeat what we've done in the past, which is we've really hung on to this culture of analog.

We still call it electronic folders and files. It's still called a wet read when we perform a quick interpretation for a radiology study.

It's called a hanging protocol for radiologists when we double click on a study and bring it up on a diagnostic monitor. We're not hanging film anymore! There's nothing wet about that film. It's not even a film anymore. So we've hung onto this culture of analog even in the way we've described the things we're doing in health IT.

I think it's really important to understand that as we look at this dawn of this new era, there's also a cultural shift that's required for us to comprehend the power of digital. The power of digital isn't just in replicating analog. It's in connecting the dots, getting to a whole different level of leveraging intelligence in our care processes.

What road map do you give clinicians who remain skeptical of using digital health tools and empowering patients?

I empathize with them. Being a clinician myself, I really do empathize with them. I'm not just saying this because we're on the same team. We're all in the same team. We're in the team that hopefully is on the side of the patient. So they have reason to be skeptical. They have been burned. They're seemingly less productive today. They're spending precious hours into the evening starting their days really early.

It's not just technology that's to be blamed. We're also in an era of doing more with less. Costs continue to escalate and reimbursement continues to decrease. There are all sorts of pressures coming at us from every which angle. But the technology and the way that it's been deployed doesn't necessarily help either. So I'm not complaining. What I'm saying is it's important for us to comprehend that it's great where we are, but we need to do so much better.

We need to give IT a chance. I think it's important for us

to work with IT and with innovators and with forward-thinking companies to really think outside the box. For clinicians, just to bring it home in terms of their experience right now, I think it was Becker's Health IT that wrote emergency department physicians spend 44% of their time entering data into the electronic medical records, clicking up to 4,000 times during a 10-hour shift. So 44% of their time is spent entering data into the EMR as opposed to, perhaps, looking at the patient or talking to them or empathizing with them or treating them right.

That's wrong. I think for clinicians, they have reasons to be skeptical, but I think it's important for them to really work with IT, leverage their background as clinicians and their knowledge and experience of what's important in providing care. They're in the business of doing the right things for patients that are in front of them, embracing the good and then embracing too this notion of simplicity, which is I think really important and sometimes a bit of a cultural shift for clinicians or anyone in health care in general.

We've traditionally been brought up with the notion that complexity is a good thing. We embrace complexity like this blanket that we hold close to us, but it's not necessarily a good thing. In fact, more often than not, if we're able to make things as simple as possible, that really takes things to a different level.

So for clinicians, technology should really be invisible. Today we've come to really tolerate technology. We're dealing with these clicks all the time, with windows that pop up all the time. We're dealing with alert fatigue all the time. So technology shouldn't really be something that we tolerate. Technology should be an enabler. Technology, at the end of the day, should be invisible. So we should get to the notion of fewer clicks and more moments because that's what health care is really about.

What story should we be telling about health care?

I speak both as a clinician and as someone who's involved in innovation in the space of health IT when I say that, for the longest time, health care has really been about curing disease and managing illness and preventing death. Nothing wrong with that. It's a very noble pursuit, and that's why I became a doctor myself. It started off many, many years ago with all sorts of different experiments and things that we tried. We tried to cure polio and invented antibiotics.

But health care shouldn't just be about not dying. Health care should really be about living. It should be about not just curing disease, but it should also be about wellness and what it means to live one's life.

This focus is important because it's really, at the end of the day, how health care continues to evolve. It shouldn't just be about the 20 minutes and that encounter in the doctor's office when you in for your annual physical. It should also be a focus on the 525,585 other minutes that year, too. What you do then or don't do then, how you're motivated then or not, really has an impact in what happens in those 20 minutes that you spend in your physician's office (or emergency department).

So health care really should be thought about as this evolving spectrum, from managing disease to curing illness, which is really important, even as we talk about population health and precision medicine. But the spectrum continues and it goes on to things like engaging consumers and behavior change and ensuring that we're able to liberate the data and empower the patients to take charge of their health and wellness.

At the end of the day, it really should be about living. It's a different focus if we think about where health care has been for the last couple of centuries versus where it needs to be in the next couple of years.

14
CREATE BEHAVIORAL CHANGE
A CONVERSATION WITH DR. MATT PATTERSON

In this chapter, you will learn why the best digital health tools usually aren't those that add more to your day; they usually allow you to be left alone to do your work. Dr. Matt Patterson is now president of AirStrip. I invited Matt on the program because I was mesmerized when his company performed a live demonstration of its AirStrip Sense4Baby digital pregnancy monitoring system at the Apple Keynote Event in September 2015. I felt like I was watching digital health innovation happening live in real time. As they showed in front of millions of streaming viewers, innovation requires a vision of what you want digital health to accomplish and how it fits within a clinical workflow. Developing a strong vision can help win over fellow clinicians and administrators simultaneously and fundamentally change care pathways.

What is your vision for the future of digital health?

With my background as a physician and also in consulting, I can tell you in a value-based reimbursement world and in a world where providers are taking on more risk and even consumers are taking on more risk, at the end of the day, the only way that you're going to be able to survive and thrive in that kind of environment is if you are creating behavior change and redesigning care pathways fundamentally from what they are today. So a doctor, a nurse, a patient, a family member, someone's behavior is going to have to improve in some meaningful way for you to drive the right outcomes.

You can do all kinds of retrospective analyses on big data and come up with the greatest conclusions ever and present a beautiful PowerPoint deck to hospital executives and say, "This is what your doctors, nurses and patients ought to be doing," but good luck going out there and actually driving their behavior change and getting them to perform in a different way that they haven't before.

Our vision around connected health is around enabling workflows and enabling decision making independent of where a clinician or consumer is across space and time. I think that's really what it's all about, and I think that that's where you're going to see the bulk of attention over the next few years.

So I think what AirStrip represents is we are in near-real time bringing in multiple disparate data sources across all vendors and landscapes inside and outside the hospital into a simple, elegant workflow that allows clinicians, patients, consumers and others to just have the perfect amount of situational awareness for their workflow to make the right next choice. What needs to happen next? And I think that that last mile is solving really what's missing in the marketplace and is a place where we can really excel.

What are the keys to driving behavior change among clinicians with digital health tools?

There are two constituents that you need to be able to have a compelling value proposition for. One is the folks who are writing your checks, and the other is the folks who you hope to be using your software or hardware. And often times the value props for those two constituents are very, very different.

Listen, I'm a doctor so I can say this. I'll tell you that doctors, by and large, really don't care about the metrics for bundled payment initiatives, or cost of care savings, or this quality metric or that quality metric, or shared savings and things like that. We honestly don't. What most doctors really want today is just to be left alone. We want to be able to do good work, to be creative and thoughtful and to take care of people. That's what we want.

But health systems are recognizing that to thrive in a value-based world and to take on risk, you need to fundamentally change the way care has been delivered, and that is a huge ask for doctors and nurses, and even patients.

So as you're thinking of innovating in a space in a hardware or software side, it's not enough to solve an economic problem or a quality problem in health care because if you don't have end users who are just violently happy about what you've created and want to use it all day every day, you're going to fail. And likewise, if you create a wonderful viral application that every doctor loves and can't live without, but yet it really doesn't solve for any important economic or quality problem in health care, it will not get adopted by health systems. You will get marginalized and commoditized.

You have to solve both of those things simultaneously and recognize that what's important for a doctor isn't necessarily what's important for the health system. As an example, consider a bundle payment initiative, something so simple as a surgical bundled payment where one of the quality metrics is a patient experience where a surgeon needs to talk to a patient before they get wheeled back from anesthesia into the OR. You would expect that's a very simple thing, everybody should get that, right? But you'd be surprised, that doesn't always happen, amazingly.

Now imagine that you're the surgeon and you have this great little technology tool that says, "The patient has arrived in anesthesia. Go see them," and you show up but the patient's not there. They're off getting a lab drawn or the patient got a lab drawn on their coagulation panel which will determine whether or not you can operate on them today. And you're going to walk up to that patient and either they're not going to be there or you're not even going to know whether or not you're operating on them and you're fumbling over what you're supposed to say. I mean, this is a disaster of a situation.

Something so simple as trying to create a tool to enable doctors and patients to just connect at the right space in the right time can be exceedingly complex when you have to take into account scheduling systems, lab systems, EMR systems, messaging systems, etc.

So the best solution in that case would be one in which the doctor gets a perfect message that says, "Patient's ready. Coags are done. Came back at this value. Ready to go. All you need to do is drop by now and say 'Hi' to them." So that is a workflow enabler where the doctor will be violently happy that that exists because now I'm not wasting my time and I'm not fumbling over something that doesn't work right. And the patients will be satisfied because it feels like everything is working seamlessly, everybody's coordinated, everybody's on the same page.

The doctor and the patient, they don't really care that the

hospital is participating in a bundled payment program and it's going to make more money and it's going to drive higher quality. They just want the seamless nature of the encounter to not be disturbed by technology. It's to be enabled by the technology. It's to be a silent partner to that. So those are the types of things and the challenges that you need to address. It seems very, very mundane when you're talking about high-tech stuff, but it's far more complicated at the operational level than most people realize.

I honestly think that physicians in particular are now facing a world where we're feeling like we're just a cog in a big machine. We went into this profession for very, very noble reasons, wanting to help people and just looking for some semblance of respect and recognition for the sacrifices that we made from an education standpoint and time standpoint to train to do what we want to do. And now we're just being asked to do a lot more for a lot less with fewer resources.

15
PATIENT ENGAGEMENT CHANGES THE GAME
A CONVERSATION WITH STERLING LANIER

In this chapter, you will learn the four pain points that an effective patient engagement platform can solve for clinicians. Sterling Lanier is CEO of Tonic. I invited Sterling on the program after having Dr. Swanson and Dr. Smith as guests and realizing that they both use Tonic as the crux of their patient engagement strategies. Sometimes the strategy isn't rocket science, but execution is a challenge. Sometimes data shows reasons for lack of engagement that you wouldn't expect, like patients needing a ride home or not being able to afford medications. And sometimes, we just need a reminder about what makes a difference for the ones in the trenches.

What types of patient engagement tools are in demand?

The environment has never been better for all types of digital health tools. We're certainly really excited about the broader push towards patient centricity and using technology to improve patient care and outcomes. I think the environment has shifted for the better.

A good example is six years ago, cloud-based systems were still a significant concern for a lot of providers and payers. The idea that you stored patient data in the cloud was still somewhat exotic. It was a significant barrier to a trial and certainly purchase. But now we just don't hear that as much anymore. Certainly security is always an issue, but folks are more open to the cloud and all the benefits it can yield in terms of cost, flexibility and efficiency.

I've certainly noticed a willingness among large enterprise health systems and payers to adopt these new tools and start to see technology as not something that's scary but something that could really drive their business forward. I think the overall idea of the cloud right now is being seen as moving from something that can hurt us to something that can really help us.

From a macro point of view, I think the current environment is great. I live and work in Palo Alto, and it feels like there's another digital health company every week finding some important vertical or niche in health care to tackle. There's certainly lots of activity on the startup side as well.

I think there are a couple of functions that folks are looking for. One, providers are requesting ways to know their patients better. When you know your patients better you can treat them better at a lower cost. This is especially important in this brave new world of value-based care, which goes to the second piece that we're certainly seeing, which is really the move towards patient-reported outcomes (PROs). It seems like you can't pick up a trade journal or any type of health care IT commentary without an article talking about PROs being a super-hot button issue.

But it's currently highly cumbersome to collect these patient-reported outcomes from patients. Again, for those of you who don't know, collecting PROs is critical because they are the new currency of value-based reimbursement models. Payers are increasingly telling a health system that they are not going to pay them for a hip surgery, for example, unless the patient says they are feeling better a month or so (or more) after the procedure. They are no longer paying for the procedure but are instead paying for the outcome. Yet today it's super clunky to collect those outcomes from the patient.

How can a patient engagement platform affect outcomes or help a provider get to know his or her patients better?

An engagement platform can affect outcomes by first getting patients to give us more information about themselves. This means pushing out surveys, forms and questionnaires electronically on a tablet, on a smartphone or on the Web—whatever is most convenient for the patient.

Second, it can also push out data back to the patient, such as a video or other patient education content. It builds that last pipe to the patient to collect data from them via surveys, forms, questionnaires, and then push out relevant data to them right at the spot.

Let's say you come in and you are filling out an intake form in a hospital or a clinic setting. It turns out that you screen in as high risk for diabetes, or you screen in as high risk for depression. An engagement platform immediately fires off an alert that tells clinicians or staff to, "Go outside right now. Or when you see this patient in the exam room shortly, you need to focus on his depression, or you need to focus on her diabetes risk."

Another example is pre-surgical triage. We have one customer who is sending out surveys 15 days in advance of a surgery. Their problem was people showing up the day of the surgery in zero shape to actually have surgery. Some portion of their patients just didn't follow the rules they were supposed to follow. The reason that this health system wanted to track it is that if patients show up prepared for surgery, they're going to have better outcomes.

So they use a tool to push out a survey 15 days before surgery, 10 days, 5 days, 4 days, 3 days, etc. If the patient answers questions a certain way and screens out for surgery, the tool will fire an alert to the surgical nurse to say, "Pick up the phone. Call Jim Smith. He seems to be having something going on here that we may need to address before surgery."

The reason I love this example is that it has an outcome that nobody perhaps was expecting in that what they found was the physical things they were trying to screen out for were not the things that impacted outcomes—such as, "Did you stop taking your anti-clotting medication before surgery?"

Instead, what impacted outcomes were social and environmental factors that they were never even being asked in the first place, such as, "Do you have a ride home? Can you afford your medications post-surgery?" In other words, elements that weren't even being tracked or asked before turned out to have the biggest impact on outcomes and readmission rates.

Hospitals get penalized if that surgery patient comes back within 30 days of being discharged. Not being able to afford your medications is going to be one reason they come right back. It's interesting how outcomes can be greatly influenced or impacted by things that perhaps aren't necessarily intuitive to us at the start.

What are the keys to patient engagement?

From my perspective, there are three keys to patient engagement, none of which are rocket science.

The first one is providing a great digital experience, whether that's through a super-fun and friendly user interface or finding other ways to surprise and delight patients. It is common sense, but it is remarkably hard to do well. How do you create a simple and intuitive process when you are oftentimes dealing with patient populations that are uncomfortable with technology or health care settings? Or take diagnosed oncology patients. Their minds are in a lot of different areas. How do we engage them in a way that gets them to focus on the information that matters most to them and their care? It's easier said than done.

You've also got to stand out through the noise of everything else going on in their life. And that's not just within health care. How do I stand apart from the noise of Facebook, from all these other cool apps they're using, Instagram, the recipe apps? How do we provide an experience that can compete with those? I think most startups are obsessed with trying to compete with other apps within health care. That's not really the way the real world works. You're competing for attention from that patient by all the other things in their life, health care-related or otherwise. That's number one.

Number two, it's really about making it convenient overall. Again, not rocket science here, but how do you do that? You've got to make it convenient for patients to either fill out the information or consume the information you're giving them, and you have to make it convenient for staff to receive and analyze the results, not having two separate systems they have to log into, for example.

For patients, we built native apps across the iPhone, iPad, and Web that allowed patients to interact in the medium and in the time that was most convenient or relevant for them. It's really about building a workflow or care pathway that is flexible enough so that it can be personalized to the patient rather than having the patient follow some rules of engagement that have somehow been dictated from above.

Third, for us it was about making that data actionable in real time. You hear a lot about patient engagement. You engage the patient, but if you're not providing feedback or giving them something in exchange for that engagement, you're eventually the boy who cried wolf. Patients are going to say, why am I engaging if I'm not seeing any type of return? So we built a system where if you tell us one thing, we're going to instantly return some type of information back to you. For example, say you take an atrial fibrillation screener. We're going to automatically return results to you and say, "Here's how you compare versus all the other 50 year old African-American men living in this zip code." It's all about giving something of meaning back to the patient in real time.

Of course, there are some cases where you don't want to show how people compare when you give them back the results, but that's just an example of how we provide meaningful feedback. "Hey, you screened in a certain way. Watch this video right now. You may be at risk for obstructive sleep apnea. Check out this video to learn some tips. Here are some things you should talk to your doctor about during your upcoming visit."

It's really about how we use that data in real time to both improve care on the clinician side and return something back to that patient for their engagement. It's focusing on how to get the right content to the right patient on the right device at the right time. It's not a rocket science idea, but it's surprisingly difficult to execute against.

What clinical pain points does a patient engagement platform overcome?

I think almost everybody working in health systems is there to provide great care. That's their main motivation. Everyone wants to create and offer a great patient experience. But the question then given the payment models becomes, what can we afford to pay for? Oftentimes just providing a great patient experience is maybe not enough to make that line item in the budget; its not a high enough ROI given all the other competing priorities in a health system. Thus, I think any patient engagement solution has to come with teeth, if you will. The teeth we define in four ways: cost, revenue, outcomes and competitive advantage.

Let's start with cost. What we try to say is that while you're providing a better patient experience, we're also going to streamline those operations so that we're going to save money at every patient interaction. Right now, every intake experience has roughly $300 to $400 of costs just in labor time of entering that data into the record. We are going to say we're going to provide a much better patient experience, but we're also going to save you all this cost, too.

The second key thing is also driving more revenue. We allow providers, for example, to offer services that have been historically challenging to provide but now they can bill for, such as the new chronic care management code from CMS, the chronic care joint replacement model from CMS and even simpler stuff like annual wellness visits. These things are tough from a requirements perspective but a patient engagement platform makes it super easy.

The third piece is certainly better outcomes. Again, the more we know about a patient, the better the care at a lower cost, or the better we can treat them at a lower cost. We can do all this through preventative care—or at least "trackable" care. We can screen your population on an ongoing basis so we can track and trend those patients over time and watch them progress. We can get you the outcome data without it being a complete pain in the rear to collect all that information and make it very easily accessible for clinicians.

The last key part that patient engagement solves is that it makes a great patient experience a huge competitive advantage. In a period of mass consolidation among providers and payers, health care organizations now need to offer an experience that patients can't get at the competing provider down the street. What you'll hear from patients who use a successful platform is that it lends the impression that their provider offers more advanced or innovative care than they can find elsewhere.

And in a value-based payment model, this becomes even more important because providers can't afford to have that patient go somewhere else. They get a fixed fee for that patient's health; if they go somewhere else, they can't track it or control it. Thus, patient engagment creates an experience where people want to stay.

So in sum it's really those four things. Yes, it's about providing a better patient experience, but it's got to have teeth, which we define as less cost, more revenue, better outcomes and an increased competitive advantage.

16
FOCUS ON CURRENT PATIENTS, NOT JUST NEW ONES
A CONVERSATION WITH SHAWN GROSS

In this chapter, you will learn that just as "health care" no longer means only check-ups, "marketing" no longer means only acquiring new patients. Shawn Gross is chief digital strategist and health care lead at White Rhino, and he discusses how hospitals benefit by shifting their focus to current patients through the next generation of mobile health experiences that have the potential to converge with clinical priorities including population health and value-based care. I invited Shawn on the program after hearing him speak on this topic at the Health Care Internet Conference (HCIC).

What is the current environment for digital health apps, and what functions are being requested?

I think of health care and provider mobile apps "1.0" as, "We've got this large institutional .org website. Help us repackage all of that content into a small form factor." What I'm seeing more and more is instead of taking a giant hospital organization's website and shrinking it down, it's creating companion experiences. It can be literally a two- or three-screen mobile app, a virtual assistant, to help get me through a procedure or maybe help in my recovery, or maybe help give me pointers and coach me for wellness and follow-up care.

Think of this idea of extending the patient's and physician's relationship outside of the hospital walls. Is there a more meaningful opportunity to use mobile apps and push notifications to nurture and build one-on-one relationships with your patients when you don't get to see them too often? Especially if you think of your primary care provider, you might see them once a year. So what kind of relationship can they have with you outside the hospital walls, and how can that be packaged into small form factor?

So it's thinking beyond just, "We've got this large website. Let's shrink it down." That's where now, I think of that world as hospital marketing Web "2.0," and we're getting more and more requests like that with some of our health care clients.

I think when it comes to requesting an appointment, or helping me pay a bill, or looking up condition and disease information, again this was all part of that first wave of what mobile apps could offer, and now in this new world, I am noticing it's much more relationship building.

So it's recognizing that I've just arrived to the hospital, maybe through the use of iBeacons, and geofencing, so extending the customer service notifications, knowing that I parked in the east garage and therefore I have to go through a few different buildings to get to my appointment. So it can include wayfinding help, customer service and follow-up care.

If I have seen my dermatologist or my gastroenterologist,

what are some of the things that they might want me to do post-procedure? Coaching me to remind me to take my medication or just drinking water may be your use case. Water can help with hundreds of ailments in the body, so your dermatologist might ask you to get into a better regimen around drinking 32 ounces of water every day. Well, wouldn't you know if you fall behind your smart phone app can send you helpful push notifications?

As a digital marketer, there are opportunities to sit with your clinical service lines, and as you map out your yearly marketing plans, shift a little bit away from the norm of search ads and landing pages and radio ads, and instead think integrated. What comes next?

It's building these one-on-one relationship or companion apps, as we like to call them, that could actually be health care marketers' new marketing program in a smartphone.

Explain how companion apps give providers a marketing advantage.

Health care marketers are trained to focus exclusively on the prospective patient. For anyone who was just recently diagnosed with cardiomyopathy, for example, maybe that's a really small population and it's even smaller if you think about the people who are savvy enough to take that diagnosis and Google it. Stop and think about the larger audiences instead that a digital marketer could help influence when they start thinking about not prospective patients, but current patients. It's a much larger audience and it's also reframing this idea of being a marketer to only people who are in need of sick care but really about offering care throughout the entire life of that patient's hospital and health care utilization, along their entire health continuum.

When you start thinking about it as that much broader spectrum, there's a world of opportunities to market to those people and create experiences, and I like to use the term "advertising without the ads" because you and I are turned off as listeners when we see advertising. Usually we know to shut down then ignore what really feels like advertising. So instead, create moments and create experiences, extensions of the health care organization that I want to be a part of that instead nurtures me, informs me, coaches and provides oversight.

It's going to feel like a digital service and it's not going to feel like an advertisement at all. It just so happens to be that the marketers at the health care organization can be the ones typically to spearhead these types of initiatives.

There are two ways we go around it but we're like kids in a candy store. We have used terms like advertising without the ads but the truth is, this new way of thinking is something we call "addictive health," and addictive in a good way.

In one patient story, the patient has been receiving care at a hospital and while there are these wonderful digital services that encapsulate and surround Mark, our fictitious patient story, they're truly just marketing programs that the hospital has decided to invest in that provide uplift, increase patient satisfaction. People wouldn't even expect these types of things from their hospitals, and they're addictive in ways because they are services that they want to continue using. They're services that they want to tell their friends and family about because they provided a great health care experience.

One of my clients at a major hospital often likes to kid around and says, "Well, when I enter work every day, I have to remember I'm leaving my digital life at the door because most hospitals don't act and don't think in digital ways." So this idea of addictive health is a new way that marketers can be working with their IT teams, with their chief experience officers or patient care service teams and really infusing marketing principles into ways that I don't think have been recently embraced by those types of departments.

Usually at most hospitals, marketing's something that's done for prospective patients and it's more in the vein of advertising, but not nurturing the existing population that is already engaging with the hospital.

So there are other people out there clamoring for more mobile health care experiences and other ways to market their health services. This concept is obviously resonating, and there are others enunciating it from different points of view.

Small little intimate moments, little experiences, again, don't have to be a lot of screens and a large development process. These can be small, two- or three-screen mobile apps or wearable apps. Another example that you'll find about addictive health is the idea of family connect. How many times have we all been in the waiting room waiting to hear how our loved one's procedure is going, also knowing that there's this large family outside of just the folks who made it that day to the waiting room? There are aunts and uncles who live on the West Coast; maybe there are relatives and family spread out throughout the country. Wouldn't it be great using the timestamp systems of the hospital's OR room?

I could get push notifications sent to this mini-private social network. It doesn't sound like marketing at all but again, it's an experience created by the hospital because they know that their patients and the family members of the patients' value digital experience. Again, going back to that statement that my client likes to say, leaving her digital life at the doorsteps of her employer every day, well, that would change in a really big way for the health care organization who wants to roll out something like family connect.

So again, it doesn't have to feel like advertising. It could be fun, addictive and something you want to share with friends.

I saw the stat that just 18% of a practice's budget is spent on marketing communications; just 18% of that budget went to actually drive 91% of all new patient acquisitions. So just think of what a small percentage of their budget was focused on current patients but that led to 90% of new business, whereas 68% was actually focused on advertising and it returned less than 1% of new business.

So I think more research in the marketplace will help health care marketers feel like they're not making a giant leap of faith but that actually some data behind focusing your marketing efforts on current patients has this halo effect, this trickle-down effect to influence new business.

How do clinicians become involved in developing companion apps?

I think that's the most important question out of all of this because I do see a lot of consumer health apps. You can go to the App Store, go to the health section and you're going to see thousands of these apps. So the logical question to be asking is, why this isn't working the way I seem to be envisioning it?

Well, that's because it's not coming from inside the hospital walls, and I think it's crucial that any health care marketer or any health care agency remember that for credibility, for sort of the litmus test of whether this is going to work or not, it must be prototyped and even developed in collaboration with clinical practices because they're on the frontlines. They know the patient experience best and they also know the pains.

So I think the answer to your question is two-fold. Whether

it's smartphone apps or wearables, I would apply the same type of thinking, and that's one, you have to use the physician group to help think it out. Is this relatable? Is this something that my patients even have a pain around? The second thing is, not to just think as a consumer marketer and create apps that already exist in the App Store.

So many miss the mark because they were too consumer focused in the sense that they didn't do their market research and didn't start with patients first as their priority audience when trying to figure out if this app was going to meet the mark.

So what do I mean by that? It means if you're a health care marketer, go talk to the pulmonology team when you create the marketing plan and actually get clear on what pains their patients have with follow-up care, or your cancer center to talk about the types of questions new patients and current patients are asking around how to live with their cancer diagnosis, health and wellness and support tips. What are the types of companion apps that could actually solve some of the challenges or dilemmas that they're facing in their life after being diagnosed with certain ailments and conditions?

Only then do I think an app that does the things that we're talking about here, creating addictive experiences, comes to life. I don't think it can be done without involving the clinical teams, and through the clinical teams you'd find that you also prototype with real patients. So I think if we sit back and just go on gut instinct and see what others have done in the marketplace and try to follow, it isn't going to create the type of work that is helpful. It's got to really come from inside the walls of a hospital, and who better to do that than a health care marketer who only has to walk down the hall or into the next building, to work with their clinicians?

17
PLAY NICE WITH THE CIO
A CONVERSATION WITH DAVID CHOU

In this chapter, you will learn why the voice of the CIO is important for digital health. David Chou is the CIO at Mercy Children's Hospital. He was formerly a CIO consultant for health care organizations around the globe. I invited him on the program because of his perspective of how clinicians and technology work together. He identifies 4 key areas of competency for today's CIO, the impact of security threats, the necessity of innovation, and winning executive buy-in by framing technology initiatives in terms of business outcomes.

What are some of the top issues facing health systems CIOs today?

When I look at the role of the CIO, there are so many things that are involved in terms of our responsibility. If I had to break them into four core components, one of components is just keeping the lights on the day-to-day operations where there's lots of organizations who have legacy infrastructures. You cannot get to just having a secure environment until you do some of that legacy infrastructure upgrade.

The second core responsibility that I see for the CIO is to innovate, right? We have to bring new ideas that are out of the box. We have to put together innovative strategies from a technology perspective that can be a competitive advantage for the organization.

The third role is to get the strategies for integration. If you have looked at what's going on in health care today, there are all kinds of mergers and acquisitions. How do you integrate a new health systems or hospital? How do you integrate new clinics that your organization may buy? So think about expansion.

For the most part, you want to be with an organization that's expanding. You never want to be in the organization that's going to get acquired. I think it's important for the CIOs to really have that integration strategy and expansion strategy in place so that when the time comes for the organization to have that discussion, you're ready to go as a true business value partner for the organization.

The last thing I think we're always struggling with, and we hear the buzzwords all the time, are analytics and big data. Organizations want to make decisions based upon data and not just make decisions based upon their experience or their intuitions. So I think that's a place where the CIO has to focus a lot to really make an organization data driven. I think that is a crucial role.

To sum it up, I will say those are the four roles that the CIOs have to play. We have to wear multiple hats now versus before. I think that should be the focus of any incoming CIO and any existing CIO that wants to provide value add for the organization.

Do you come across any common misconceptions about the role of the CIO?

Definitely. They've used the CIO role as a utility and that's traditionally how it has been in the past. The CIO is a pretty new role. It probably came about in the '90s or 2000s. But prior to that, even in my career I recall when there was not a CIO role. There was a department that we called data processing. That was pretty much the folks that took care of anything related to technology.

It's been an expense which is why lots of organizations do have the CIOs reporting to the CFOs. I think that is still the image of the CIO and the technology department. So it's really up to the leader to change that image. Ultimately, we have to become a business leader versus just a pure technology leader.

When a clinician is interested in innovation, or they have an idea or at the very least they want to engage with patients and they want to use digital health tools and they hear about new tools that are coming out—it might be an app or an entire engagement platform—how does a CIO support clinicians in that case?

I think number one, we have to listen to those ideas and we have to be engaged with what's out there in the market. Traditionally, the CIOs have always said no to anything that doesn't come out from their own team or group. I think that has always set a bad taste in the end user's mouth, and that has to change.

For example, it's not okay to have a device working better at your house than your corporate environment. If your iPhone is faster than your PC or laptop at your work, that is not acceptable. So I think we as consumers are getting smarter, meaning your employees are getting smarter as well. They have the latest and greatest at their home, and they're going to want to use that type of device at the work environment. They're going to want the same convenience factor.

It's really up to the CIOs to, number one, listen. Number two, understanding the experience that the end users want. End users could be your employees, the nursing staff, clinicians and the patients. So it's really understanding how to create that experience utilizing the tools that may be different. It doesn't always have to be something that's already out there from the existing market.

I think CIOs really have to see the latest and greatest and explore other avenues in terms of innovation. A lot of that goes to listening. You really have to listen. You have to be open to engaging, take valuable inputs, see how you can make that work and find that balance.

How can health IT vendors support your mission as the CIO?

You have to have a partnership. I think vendors play a strong role. If you talk about any EMR rollout or any huge projects, the CIO's teams cannot function without a good partnership.

I think it's really up to the vendors to support that. I leave it on the vendors to create that strategy at times as well. You have to stay engaged with them in terms of where they are focusing on, where are they headed the next two or three years. Make sure that's in line with your organization's business objectives.

I will say that's a really strong partnership that needs to exist. The advice should be if they really want to have a seat at the table and be that true partner, they have to understand the business problem versus making a quick sale. I've seen lots of vendors out there who are just good at making a quick sale, and the next time they call you is probably three years later when your renewal is due or when it's time for a refresh. Those are not considered partners.

The partners are the ones who are going to be with you every step of the way. They're going to provide some business insight, some valuable input. That's what I would recommend to vendors in terms of the engagement with the CIOs to be able to provide value. Otherwise, it's very transactional.

What else would you like to share with the health care community?

Well I would say if you look at the grand scheme of things, we have gone a long way in the last eight years. Prior to Meaningful Use, we were not electronic. So when I look at the grand scheme of things coming from a paper environment, where the majority of health care organizations were to being mostly electronic these days within eight to nine years, that's a major feat, a major accomplishment.

If we look at the grand scheme of things here, we really have come a long way. But when you start thinking about the day to day, the year to year, what we have done differently, what we have changed, it really feels like we haven't done much. But when you look at the grand scheme of things, I think that the entire health care vertical has come a long way. We just have to find a way to keep that momentum going and maybe leapfrog a few years so that we could get to where we want to be in our mindset.

18
OWN YOUR CAREER
A CONVERSATION WITH SUE SCHADE

In this chapter, you will learn how to determine if an EHR rollout is successful, the value of the CMIO and the difference between problems and solutions. Sue Schade is a founding adviser at Next Wave Health Advisors, a small advisory services firm of some of the leading CIOs in the country. I invited Sue on the program after hearing her speak at a #HealthITChicks panel discussion at HIMSS in March 2016. In addition to her insights as a CIO and CMIO consultant, Sue gives valuable advice for owning your career and breaking down gender barriers in a traditionally male-dominated field.

Is there an average time for an EHR implementation, and how do you determine whether it is successful?

The average timeframe is going to vary based on the size of your organization, what you're moving off of and on to, and the product that you're using.

As far as how you measure success, various articles have been written on this. You don't have people saying, "Let's go back. Let's just throw it out entirely." You just don't hear that. Clinicians accept that this is where we are at this point in time.

But you want fewer clicks and streamlined workflows. You want a high degree of integration so that there is easy access to all the information on the patient, between the inpatient and outpatient setting for all specialties. Then you need to be able to take it to that next layer of health information exchanges within your state or within your region.

You want to be able to get the information that another provider organization—even a competitor—may have on your patient to have a complete picture of that patient's health history.

What is the role of the CMIO?

The Chief Medical Information Officer is a very important partner to the CIO. I'm not hearing of very many models where the CMIO reports to the CIO. Especially in larger organizations, the CMIO often reports to a Chief Quality Officer or to the Chief Medical Officer, with a close relationship with the CIO, or possibly a dotted line to the CIO. I look at it as a true partnership.

I have come to appreciate CMIOs, having worked with a couple of solid ones now. The importance of their clinical knowledge, their clinical background, their relationships with the clinicians, the respect and credibility that they have with clinicians makes a huge difference when you are trying to get something done, when you're rolling out something new, when you're trying to understand the workflows and the clinician needs, or quite frankly, when you've got problems and issues, and you need that clinician to be able to talk to the clinical leaders.

They oftentimes can do that more effectively than the technical folks within IT.

What are some of the obstacles keeping telehealth from being adopted more widely?

The reimbursement models vary state to state in terms of whether telemedicine is covered or not. I think you'll also run into very different needs and models depending on the state, region, and provider organization that you're in.

Some of the more successful deployments are in areas where there's a main academic medical center hub that's serving a broad rural population, and they have figured out what that model needs to look like and been able to deploy successfully.

Others in more urban areas are still trying to answer the question of whether you are basically making it more convenient for the patient who doesn't need to get in traffic and find a place to park for a very simple visit. It really depends on the area that you're in, what the needs of that population are and then, of course, the reimbursement models.

But I don't think it's really technology that is the obstacle at this point. It's a matter of figuring out what the requirements are, the workflow and then the financial framework for it.

You spoke at the #HealthITChicks panel discussion at HIMSS and gave some great career advice in general. What career advice do you have for women in health IT?

This may not be specific to women in health IT, but broadly. I'll come back to women in health IT later.

First and foremost, I think you have to develop a sense of confidence in yourself that, even when you don't feel it, you somehow have to draw on an inner strength and project confidence.

I think it's really important that you develop a network and find someone that you would like to have as your role model and potentially mentor you. It's really important to recognize that you own your own career. People aren't going to hand things to you or do things for you necessarily. You own it. You have to make the choices at the right time for yourself.

I would also emphasize, don't take crap! Don't put up with stuff that you know is just wrong. You've got to be an advocate for yourself and speak up.

As far as women in IT, it's an area that I've written about in my weekly blog as well as spoken about quite a bit in the past year. There is a need to get more women and girls, starting young, interested in technology in the STEM field: science, technology, engineering and math.

I'm trying to encourage leaders to support that and find ways to promote it and actively encourage young girls to go into those fields. They are lagging way behind.

How can men and women collaborate to break down some of the gender barriers in health care?

Well, showing up is a start. It was mostly women in that audience [at HIMSS] and there were a number of men, so I think just recognizing that there are needs in this area is a step.

Especially if you're in management roles, you really need to look at the HR policies within your organization and how you can influence them or how they support both men and women moving ahead in their career in terms of balancing their family lives with their careers. Flexibility in the workplace for both men and women is important.

We can look at the culture we want to create and sustain in being supportive of women, but really supportive of all workers, and look at whether our policies also create that same supportive and flexible environment. So those would be two ways.

In summary, if you let something go and say, "Oh, that's just how it always is," that's the same as contributing to letting that behavior continue. That's what we've got to break away from. We need to recognize first and foremost, that there are things being said, and that things won't change unless there's an active participation in it.

19
COLLABORATION IS THE NEW SUCCESS
A CONVERSATION WITH NICK ADKINS

In this chapter, we wrap up with a final thought about collaboration in health. Nick Adkins is the kilt-wearing man responsible for the #pinksocks trend that started at HIMSS 2015. (Check out the pinksocks tribe at pinksocks.life.) I invited him on the program because he is an advocate for working together across all areas of health care. Applying this concept to developing new products is the new path to success.

What advice do you have for trying to develop a digital health product?

I say you better have a patient, a nurse, a doctor, anybody else in the workflow chain, you should have them all sitting at the table, looking at the whiteboard, each with a marker in their hand so they can go up and write stuff on the board that's input on the design process.

Unfortunately what happens a lot of times is a doctor has a great idea, or a business guy has a great idea. They don't really talk together, and so one says, "Oh. This is all going to be clinical, clinical, clinical," and sometimes the business guy says, "No. This is the business thing. It's all business, business, business," and those scenarios aren't about involving everyone.

Involve everyone who is going to use this thing, from the doctor, the patient, to the nurse, the lab tech, to the patient's mom and dad, the brother and sister and the pharmacist and everyone that may need to use this. Everyone needs to be involved in the very beginning of the design process.

I think it's the bigger thought, this realization that health care isn't just during a particular point in time, that it really is this spectrum that's going on all the time, and it's not just physicians.

There are many others that fall into that clinician bucket that are involved, one way or the other, and they would all have something to do with a lot of products like this.

You routinely see me tweet the hashtag #EinPower. "Ein" is also the German word for "one." Ein is also the name of our data dog/mascot. When I hashtag something with "#EinPower," it means "the power of one" or in other words, "we're all in this together," and that's how this is.

Health care and the evolution of where it's going today, not some far-off, five-year timeline, but what's happening today, is succeeding because of "We're all in this together." The archaic days of old silos and domains and kingdoms and fiefdoms—those days are over. They're gone. We all have to work together. It's a collaborative effort. The days of secrets and not sharing information, they're gone. We have to be working together to pull this off for all of us.

What advice would you give to clinicians who are willing to adopt digital health tools but don't know where to start?

You'd be surprised what your patients are going to tell you. You're going to start seeing more consumers walking into their doctors, showing their doctors really cool new apps that the doctors weren't even aware of. So I'd say, listen to what your patients are showing you and what apps they have on their phones that they want to use.

I think a lot of the big facilities have some super-cool apps that they've already spun up and rolled out and are rolling out right now as we speak. I think clinicians who've got great tech teams wrapped around them have vetted a lot of really good stuff.

I would show up and participate and get my voice and involvement and become part of that review process at those facilities if I were a provider. I would not sit back and be passive. I'd be actively involved in wanting to know what the facility is rolling out, from a tech standpoint, to get in my hands to use and facilitate effective communication with my patients.

ABOUT THE AUTHOR

Jared Johnson is a digital health evangelist, thought leader and the digital marketing manager for Phoenix Children's Hospital. Onalytica listed him as a #DigitalHealth Top 100 Influencer, and his peers named him to the #HIT100. He is a speaker, blogger and host of the Health IT Marketer Podcast.

Jared is on a mission to improve patient care through digital health after witnessing loved ones pass away partially due to a lack of care coordination. He speaks to groups nationwide about the impact of digital health. His other side hustle is music, having released four solo piano albums and a sheet music blog. A native Texan, he now lives in Arizona with his wife and their four young children.

www.ingramcontent.com/pod-product-compliance
Lightning Source LLC
Chambersburg PA
CBHW070242190526
45169CB00001B/273